www.harcourtinternational.com

Bringing you products from all Harcourt Health Sciences
companies including Baillière Tindall, Churchill Livingstone,
Mosby and W.B. Saunders

- ▶ **Browse** for latest information on new books, journals and electronic products

- ▶ **Search** for information on over 20 000 published titles with full product information including tables of contents and sample chapters

- ▶ **Keep up to date** with our extensive publishing programme in your field by registering with eAlert or requesting postal updates

- ▶ **Secure online ordering** with prompt delivery, as well as full contact details to order by phone, fax or post

- ▶ **News** of special features and promotions

If you are based in the following countries, please visit the
country-specific site to receive full details of product
availability and local ordering information

USA: www.harcourthealth.com

Canada: www.harcourtcanada.com

Australia: www.harcourt.com.au

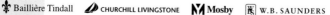

Baillière Tindall   CHURCHILL LIVINGSTONE   Mosby   W.B. SAUNDERS

CHURCHILL'S POCKETBOOK OF
Toxicology

Commissioning Editor: Timothy Horne
Project Development Manager: Fiona Conn
Project Manager: Frances Affleck
Designer: Erik Bigland

CHURCHILL'S POCKETBOOK OF
Toxicology

Alison L. Jones
BSc (Hons), MD, FRCPE
Consultant Physician and Medical Toxicologist,
Honorary Senior Lecturer in Clinical Pharmacology,
National Poisons Information Service,
Guy's and St Thomas' NHS Trust,
London, UK

Paul I. Dargan
MRCP(UK)
Registrar in Toxicology,
National Poisons Information Service,
Guy's and St Thomas' NHS Trust,
London, UK

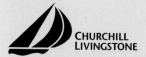

CHURCHILL LIVINGSTONE

EDINBURGH LONDON NEW YORK
PHILADELPHIA ST LOUIS SYDNEY TORONTO 2001

CHURCHILL LIVINGSTONE
An imprint of Harcourt Publishers Limited

First published 2001

ISBN 0443064768

British Library Cataloguing in Publication Data
A catalogue record for this book is available from the
British Library

Library of Congress Cataloging in Publication Data
A catalog record for this book is available from the
Library of Congress

Note
Medical knowledge is constantly changing. As new
information becomes available, changes in treatment,
procedures, equipment and the use of drugs become
necessary. The authors and the publishers have taken
care to ensure that the information given in this text
is accurate and up-to-date. However, readers are
strongly advised to confirm that the information,
especially with regard to drug usage, complies with
the latest legislation and standards of practice.

Printed in China

Contents

Preface

Clinical toxicology is the study of the exposure of humans to excessive doses of drugs or other substances. Acute poisoning remains one of the commonest medical emergencies, accounting for 10–20% of hospital admissions for general medicine.

This book has been designed as a practical, pragmatic guide to help doctors and nurses identify the type and severity of poisoning and appropriately manage patients poisoned by a wide variety of toxins. It is not designed to provide a mechanistic explanation of poisoning, for which there are much larger reference books available, but a practical hands-on guide, with warnings about potential pitfalls in diagnosis and management. The first section gives a breakdown of the basic principles of care of poisoned patients, including gut decontamination, the use of antidotes, and management of complications associated with poisoning such as arrhythmias and seizures. This is followed by two sections that provide practical management guidelines for all common poisons.

Both authors are actively involved in the care of poisoned patients and acute medical inpatients and outpatients at Guy's and St Thomas' hospitals, as well as providing telephone advice for doctors and nurses on the treatment of patients on behalf of the National Poisons Information Service. This book contains all the recent guidelines on the care of poisoned patients published by the European Association of Poisons Centres and Clinical Toxicologists and the American Academy of Clinical Toxicology. However, clinical toxicology is very much an experience-based specialty, as much of the literature is individual case reports rather than controlled studies. No book or database can substitute for advice from clinical toxicologists, and the reader is encouraged to make referrals to poisons centres in the event of serious poisoning or where unusual complications occur.

A.J. 2001
P.D.

Acknowledgements

AJ and PD would gratefully like to acknowledge the contribution of the information officers at the NPIS (London) Centre to the preparation of some of the material in this book.

Abbreviations

2,4-D	2,4-dichlorophenoxyacetic acid
4-MP	4-methylpyrazole
ABG	arterial blood gas
ACE	angiotensin converting enzyme
AChE	acetylcholinesterase
AIDS	acquired immune deficiency syndrome
ALT	alanine aminotransferase
ARDS	acute respiratory distress syndrome
AST	aspartate aminotransferase
AXR	abdominal X-ray
BAL	British anti-lewsite
BP	blood pressure
CK	creatinine kinase
CNS	central nervous system
COPD	chronic obstructive pulmonary disease
CPAP	continuous positive airway pressure
CVP	central venous pressure
DMPS	2,3-dimercapto-1-propanesulphonate
DMSA	2,3-dimercaptosuccinic acid
ECG	electrocardiogram
EDTA	sodium calcium edetate
EEG	electroencephalogram
FBC	full blood count
G-6-PD	glucose-6-phosphate dehydrogenase
GCS	Glasgow Coma Scale
GHB	gammahydroxybutyric acid
GI	gastrointestinal
HIV	human immunodeficiency virus
INR	international normalised ratio
IU	international unit
LSD	lysergic acid diethylamide
MABP	mean arterial blood pressure
MAOI	monoamine-oxidase inhibitor
MDAC	multiple-dose activated charcoal
MDA	3,4-methylene-dioxyamphetamine
MDEA	3,4-methylene-dioxyethylamphetamine
MDMA	3,4-methylene-dioxymethamphetamine
MI	myocardial infarction
NSAID	non-steroidal anti-inflammatory drug
P2S	pralidoxine
PEEP	positive end expiratory pressure
PSS	poisons severity score

PT	prothrombin time		**TCA**	tricyclic antidepressant
SSRI	selective serotonin re-uptake inhibitor		**VF**	ventricular fibrillation
SVT	supraventricular tachycardia		**VT**	ventricular tachycardia
			WBI	whole bowel irrigation

BASIC PRINCIPLES

ASSESSING THE PATIENT

ABC

First ensure that:

- the **A**irway is clear
- the patient is **B**reathing adequately
- the **C**irculation is not compromised.

If the patient is alert and has a stable circulation, proceed to take a history and examine the patient, unless immediate eye or skin decontamination is required.

Taking a history

In the vast majority of cases, the diagnosis of acute poisoning is reached from the history given by the patient. However, doctors need to be aware that patients may not always furnish them with the correct answer. This may be because they do not always know what they have taken, not least because they may have been under the influence of alcohol or the drug itself at the time of ingestion or when giving you a history. A few patients deliberately mislead doctors but in our experience this is very rare, except perhaps in the drug abuser population.

Full details of how many and what type of substance has been taken must be recorded, as well as timing of ingestion or exposure. Whether the drugs belonged to the patient or a friend or relative and the source (i.e. over the counter, prescription, street, etc.) is important in future prevention of poisoning. The nature of any drug taken can be corroborated or identified from descriptions of tablets or remaining pills (or their packets/bottles) by use of drug identification software (e.g. TICTAC), which can be accessed by many pharmacy departments and all National Poisons Information Service centres in the UK.

Ask the patient why the overdose was taken and take time to listen to the explanation. Often reasons include relationship difficulties, work or school-related difficulties, problems of addiction, psychiatric illness or bereavement. Beware of those claiming an 'accidental overdose'. Whilst this clearly can occur, e.g. paracetamol poisoning after toothache, in general all patients presenting with poisoning should undergo psychiatric evaluation.

Details of the past medical history should be recorded. In particular a history of asthma, jaundice, drug abuse (by which routes), head injury, epilepsy, cardiovascular problems and previous psychiatric history or self-harm should be taken. It is important to ask about allergies and alcohol history. Family problems and social history are very important but often missed out in undue haste to clerk the patient.

The clinical examination

A standard clinical examination should be carried out on every poisoned patient. In addition, particular care should be taken to look for needle marks or previous evidence of self-harm, e.g. razor marks on forearms. The weight of the patient is often critical in determining if toxicity is likely to occur given the dose ingested and for appropriate therapy to be calculated correctly, e.g. the N-acetylcysteine dose for paracetamol poisoning.

The Glasgow Coma Scale (Table 1.1) is the most frequently used in the assessment of the degree of impaired consciousness, though remarkably it has never been validated for use in poisoned patients.

TABLE 1.1   The Glasgow Coma Scale

	Score
Eye opening:	
Spontaneously	4
To speech	3
To pain	2
None	1
Best verbal response:	
Orientated	5
Confused	4
Inappropriate words	3
Incomprehensible sounds	2
None	1
Best motor responses:	
Obeys commands	6
Localisation to pain	5
Normal flexion to pain	4
Spastic flexion	3
Extension to pain	2
None	1
Max score = 15; Min score = 3	

> Warning! Beware patients feigning unconsciousness.
> Remember to record the *best* response for the GCS.

When patients are unconscious and no history is available, the diagnosis of poisoning depends on exclusion of other causes of coma (such as meningitis or encephalitis, trauma, subarachnoid haemorrhage, intracranial bleeds, subdural and extradural haematomas, hypoglycaemia, diabetic ketoacidosis, uraemia, encephalopathy) and consideration of circumstantial evidence.

Examination findings such as pupil size, respiratory rate and heart rate may support the diagnosis in an unconscious patient, but on their own may merely help to narrow down the potential list of toxins (Table 1.2).

A number of toxins have a characteristic odour (Table 1.3). However, the odour may be subtle and the ability to smell the odour may vary (e.g. only about 50% of the general population can smell the 'bitter almond' odour of cyanide).

TABLE 1.2 Clinical features which point to the substance responsible for poisoning in an unconscious or unwell patient

Clinical feature	Possible cause
Pinpoint pupils, reduced respiratory rate	• Opioids • Cholinesterase inhibitors (organophosphorus or carbamate insecticides) • Clonidine • Phenothiazines
Cyanosis	Any CNS depressant or agent causing methaemoglobinaemia
Needle tracks, pinpoint pupils, reduced respiratory rate	i.v. opioids
Dilated pupils or mid-point pupils, reduced respiratory rate	Benzodiazepines
Dilated pupils, tachycardia	• Tricyclic antidepressants – dry mouth, warm peripheries, may also be twitchy or have seizures • Amphetamines, ecstasy, cocaine – may also be hallucinating or agitated • Anticholinergic drugs such as benzhexol, benztropine – may also have hyperreflexia and myoclonus • Antihistamines – may also be drowsy
Increased salivation	Organophosphorus or carbamate insecticides
Cerebellar signs; nystagmus, ataxia	• Anticonvulsants (particularly phenytoin, carbamazepine) • Alcohol
Extrapyramidal signs	• Phenothiazines • Haloperidol • Metoclopramide
Seizures	Many drugs can cause seizures in overdose – common agents include: • Tricyclic antidepressants • Theophylline • Antihistamines • Anticonvulsants • Non-steroidal drugs • Phenothiazines • Isoniazid
Hyperthermia	• Amphetamines, ecstasy, cocaine (also hypertension, tachycardia, agitation, rhabdomyolysis) • Neuroleptic malignant syndrome (also confusion, fluctuating consciousness, rigidity, tremor, autonomic instability, sweating, rhabdomyolysis) • Serotonin syndrome (also agitation, clonus, tremor, hyperreflexia, sweating, tachycardia) • Salicylates including aspirin (also tachycardia, metabolic acidosis, restlessness, hyperventilation)

(Contd.)

TABLE 1.2 (Continued)

Clinical feature	Possible cause
Hyperthermia	● Lithium ● Tricyclic antidepressants, anticholinergics, antihistamines
Bradycardia	● Beta-blockers ● Calcium antagonists (not dihydropyridines) ● Digoxin ● Opioids ● Organophosphorus insecticides ● Centrally acting alpha agonists e.g. clonidine
Abdominal cramps, diarrhoea, tachycardia, restlessness, hallucinations	Withdrawal from: ● Alcohol ● Benzodiazepines ● Opioids

TABLE 1.3 Characteristic odour of toxins

Odour	Cause
Acetone	Isopropyl alcohol, acetone
Bitter almonds	Cyanide
Garlic	Arsenic, selenium, thallium
Rotten eggs	Hydrogen sulphide, mercaptans
Wintergreen	Methyl-salicylate

TABLE 1.4 Urine colour caused by certain toxins

Urine colour	Cause
Green or blue	Methylene blue, e.g. fish tank tablets
Orange or orange-red	Rifampicin Iron (especially after desferrioxamine has been started)
Grey-black	Phenols, cresols
Opaque appearance which settles on standing	Primidone crystals
Brown	Myoglobinuria (i.e. rhabdomyolysis) Haemoglobinuria

Rarely, the colour of the urine (Table 1.4) may give a diagnostic clue as to what has been taken.

Brief assessment of suicidal intent

In order to decide on the most appropriate placement and staffing ratio for a self-poisoned patient, an assessment of suicidal intent must be made. Formal psychiatric evaluation is often undertaken the next day after the effects of

TABLE 1.5 Beck's scoring system

Parameter	Scoring	Beck 's score (add up all those relevant below)
0	Isolation	Someone present
1		Someone nearby or in vocal contact
2		No-one nearby or in visual/vocal contact
0	Timing	Intervention probable
1		Intervention not likely
2		Intervention highly unlikely
0	Precautions against discovery or interruption	None
1		Passive precautions (avoiding others but doing nothing to prevent intervention)
2		Active precautions, e.g. locking door
0	Acting to gain help after the attempt	Notified potential helper regarding the attempt
1		Contacted but did not specifically notify helper regarding the attempt
2		Did not contact or notify helper
0	Final acts in anticipation of death	None
1		Thought about or made some arrangement
2		Definite plans made, e.g. changing will
0	Active preparation for attempt	None
1		Minimal
2		Extensive
0	Suicide note	None
1		Note written but torn up or thought about
2		Note present
0	Overt communication of intent before attempt	None
1		Equivocal communication
2		Unequivocal communication

sedative agents etc. have worn off, but an initial clinical assessment using the Beck's depression scale (Table 1.5) or similar may be valuable. If the sum of all the scores for each parameter is greater than 4, e.g. suicide note left and no-one likely to find patient after the overdose, it indicates significant suicidal intent.

Interpretation of laboratory results

Full analytical toxicology services are available in only a few centres and a 'toxicology screen' rarely influences initial inpatient management. A toxicology screen can be helpful in confirming the diagnosis in a small subset of patients and can be important if homicide, assault or child abuse is suspected. When the patient is first seen in A&E a 50 ml sample of urine and 10 ml sample of serum should be saved in the fridge – it is always better to take a sample that turns out not to be needed than to think of it the next day when it may be too late.

Interpretation of blood gases
It is helpful to consider the following when interpreting ABG results:

- What is the inspired oxygen gradient? Look at the PaO_2? What is the A-a gradient?
- Look at the pH – is the patient acidaemic (pH < 7.35) or alkalaemic (pH > 7.45)?
- Look at the pCO_2. Is it low, normal or high? If the pCO_2 is consistent with the change in pH, the primary abnormality is respiratory.
- If the pCO_2 is normal or does not explain the abnormality in pH, look at the base deficit/excess. If the base deficit/excess is consistent with the abnormality in pH then the primary abnormality is metabolic.

Respiratory acidosis: *pH < 7.3, pCO_2 > 5.6 kPa.* Hypoventilation from any cause results in retention of CO_2 and respiratory acidosis. Such a picture may occur in any overdose with CNS depressant drugs. With a chronic respiratory acidosis, the compensation that occurs is a rise in the bicarbonate.

Respiratory alkalosis: *pH > 7.45, pCO_2 < 4.7 kPa.* Hyperventilation and respiratory alkalosis may occur in response to hypoxia, drugs and CNS injury. The classical drug causing this is aspirin (p. 80).

Metabolic alkalosis: *pH > 7.45, Bicarbonate > 30 mmol/L.* This is uncommon in poisoning. It may result from the loss of acid or rarely from excess administration of alkali.

Metabolic acidosis: *pH < 7.35, Bicarbonate < 24 mmol/L, Base Deficit < −3.* (Compensation is pCO_2 < 4.7 kPa.) This is very common in poisoning. If severe, one should be alert to the possibility of poisoning by ethanol, methanol or ethylene glycol (pp. 110, 112). Calculation of the anion and osmolal gaps can be helpful in differentiating the cause of a toxic metabolic acidosis.

The anion gap. When reduction of plasma bicarbonate is marked, the anion gap should be calculated from:

Anion Gap $= ([Na^+] + [K^+]) - ([Cl^-] + [HCO_3^-])$

It is normally 12 ± 2. Many poisons cause a high anion gap metabolic acidosis, these include ethanol, methanol, ethylene glycol, metformin, cyanide, isoniazid and salicylates.

This list can be narrowed down further by also measuring the osmolal gap.

The osmolal gap. The osmolal gap is the difference between the laboratory measured osmolality (O_m) and the calculated osmolality (O_c). The formula for calculated osmolality is:

$O_c = 2(Na^+ + K^+) + Urea + Glucose$

The osmolal gap is normally less than 10. Common toxic causes of a raised osmolal gap include ethanol, methanol, isopropanol and ethylene glycol.

Drug levels

Drug levels in blood may be of value in patients with altered consciousness (drugs of abuse, paracetamol), iron poisoning, lithium poisoning, paracetamol and salicylate poisoning (see under specific drug).

GUIDELINES FOR GUT DECONTAMINATION

The majority of patients who present after an overdose require only meticulous supportive care. However, it is important that patients are observed closely for signs of deterioration. Overall the mortality from acute poisoning is less than 1% and it is in patients who have taken significant overdoses that further measures such as gastric decontamination and measures to increase elimination may be required.

Gut decontamination procedures include gastric lavage, ipecac induced emesis, activated charcoal and whole bowel irrigation. These procedures should only be used in patients who untreated would risk serious poisoning, as they can be associated with complications.

Ipecacuanha

Ipecacuanha (ipecac) induced emesis is no longer recommended because it is ineffective at removing significant quantities of poisons from the stomach and the vomiting it produces can confuse the clinical picture and limits the use of activated charcoal.

Further reading

American Academy of Clinical Toxicology; European Association of Poison Control Centres and Clinical Toxicologists. Position statement: Ipecac syrup. Clin Tox 1997; 35: 699–709.

Gastric lavage

Gastric lavage (stomach washout) should only be undertaken if the patient has ingested a potentially life-threatening amount of a poison and presents within *1 hour* of the ingestion. If performed later than this the amount of poison removed is insignificant and lavage can actually make the situation worse by pushing unabsorbed poison into the small intestine. Always ensure that the patient's airway is adequately protected before gastric lavage. (See Table 1.6)

TABLE 1.6 When gastric lavage should *not* be used	
Contraindication to lavage	Reason
After ingestion of hydrocarbons (e.g. white spirit, petrol, paraffin, etc.)	Risk of aspiration pneumonitis
After ingestion of corrosives (e.g. acids, alkalis, bleach, oven cleaner etc.)	Risk of gut perforation and aspiration of corrosives into the lung
If the airway cannot be protected	Risk of aspiration
As a punitive measure	As well as being unethical, there is no evidence that it prevents subsequent self poisoning

Prior to the procedure check that oxygen and powerful suction equipment is present and working. You will need KY jelly, a disposable gastric lavage tube (14 mm diameter (36–40 F) in adults), a bucket, a jug of between 250–500 ml capacity and protective clothes or covering and gloves for the staff. At least two members of staff should be present. Because of the risk of hypoxia and arrhythmias, it is advisable to monitor a patient with an oxygen saturation probe during the procedure. If gastric lavage is indicated and the patient is drowsy and unable to protect his airway, intubate with a cuffed endotracheal tube prior to gastric lavage.

The person performing the procedure should wear gloves, apron and boots. The patient should be lying in the left lateral position. The foot of the bed or trolley should be raised by 20 cm. The disposable gastric lavage tube is next lubricated with KY jelly and passed by asking the patient to swallow gently. Ensure it is not passed into the airway by keeping the head forward in a flexed position. Confirm the end of the tube is in the stomach by aspirating or blowing air in and auscultating over the stomach. Put the end of the tube into the bucket, which is held below the level of the patient, and allow the stomach contents to siphon off.

Next, connect the tube to a large funnel (using a rubber or plastic hose) and pour 300–400 ml aliquots of tepid tap water into the stomach and siphon off again by gravity or active suction. Repeat the procedure until the returning fluid is clear of particles. It may be helpful to adjust the position of the patient slightly to allow water to reach all parts of the stomach.

Once the returning fluid is clear give activated charcoal (50 g adults, 1 g/kg children) down the tube (if the toxin is adsorbed to charcoal) and then withdraw the tube taking care to occlude it completely with the fingers so fluid left in the tube does not pour into the pharynx as the tube is withdrawn. Suction may then be required to clear the oropharynx further.

TABLE 1.7   Gastric lavage complications and how to avoid them

Complication	Solution
Oesophageal rupture	Do not use force to pass the tube
Aspiration pneumonitis	Care with water and contents, adequate airway protection, suction apparatus must be present and working
Lipoid pneumonia	Do not wash out petroleum distillates, e.g. paraffin, petrol, furniture polishes
Hypoxia	Monitor oxygen saturation, give supplemental oxygen via nasal prongs

Warning! Gastric lavage should never be undertaken as a punitive procedure. Do not wash out patients beyond 1 hour after ingestion.
Beware of worsening cardiovascular status during lavage where hypoxia and pushing the contents beyond the pylorus (which increases absorption) cause sudden deterioration, particularly with tricyclic antidepressants.
Gastric lavage against a patient's wishes constitutes assault.

Further reading
American Academy of Clinical Toxicology; European Association of Poison Control Centres and Clinical Toxicologists. Position statement: Gastric lavage. Clin Tox 1997; 35: 711–719.

Jorens PG, Joosens EJ, Nagler JM. Changes in arterial oxygen tension after gastric lavage for drug overdose. Hum Exp Toxicol 1991; 10: 221–224.

Saetta JP, March S, Gaunt ME et al. Gastric emptying procedures in the self-poisoned patient: are we forcing gastric content beyond the pylorus? J R Soc Med 1991; 84: 272–276.

Activated charcoal
Activated charcoal is black slurry, which owing to its large surface area is highly effective at adsorbing many toxins. It is highly effective at adsorbing most poisons with a few exceptions owing to its large surface area and porous structure.

Agents not adsorbed by activated charcoal:

- Metal salts, e.g. iron, lithium, potassium.
- Alcohols, e.g. ethanol, ethylene glycol, methanol.
- Other agents, e.g. cyanide, hydrocarbons, solvents, acids, alkalis, fluoride.

It should be given to all patients who present within *1 hour* of ingestion of a potentially toxic amount of poison which binds to charcoal. In certain circumstances it may be warranted to give activated charcoal more than 1 hour after ingestion, e.g. following an exceptionally large overdose of a substance that slows gastric emptying (e.g. tricyclic antidepressant, opioid) providing the airway is protected.

Activated charcoal can be given via a nasogastric tube if the patient will not swallow activated charcoal or has a reduced level of consciousness. The airway must be adequately protected before activated charcoal is given.

Repeated doses of activated charcoal are also effective at increasing the elimination of some poisons from the body (see p. 13).

Contraindications to administration of activated charcoal:

- More than 1 hour since ingestion.
- Substance not bound to charcoal (see above).
- Airway cannot be protected.
- Oral antidote is given.

Available formulations of activated charcoal vary from one country to another. Medicoal®in the UK is an effervescent preparation containing sodium citrate and povidone and must be mixed with water before use. Carbomix®comes in ready to use containers, to which water must be added. Liquichar®and Actidose aqua®come as ready prepared mixtures.

Activated charcoal is given in 50 g doses for adults and 1 g/kg for children. It commonly causes vomiting and so if a patient is vomiting or nauseated prior to its administration, an antiemetic should be given (p. 23). The dose for multiple-dose charcoal is 50 g 4-hourly for an adult (see p. 13 for the indication for multiple-dose activated charcoal). Sometimes,

TABLE 1.8   Activated charcoal complications and how to avoid them

Complication	Solution
Medicoal causes diarrhoea	Could be regarded as a therapeutic advantage in some cases
Other charcoals cause constipation and rarely bezoars and even intestinal obstruction	Give a purgative when more than one dose of charcoal is given
Adsorption of oral antidotes	Do not give charcoal and oral antidote
Aspiration pneumonitis	Protect the airway, care in administration to unconscious patients

for example in salicylate poisoning, charcoal may be given 2-hourly to limit absorption of the drug.

> Warning! Do not add flavouring or colouring agents to charcoals as they reduce its adsorptive power. For the same reason ice cream should not be given with charcoal.

Further reading

American Academy of Clinical Toxicology; European Association of Poison Control Centres and Clinical Toxicologists. Position statement: Single-dose activated charcoal. Clin Tox 1997; 35: 721–741.

Menzies DG, Busuttil A, Prescott LF. Fatal pulmonary aspiration of oral activated charcoal. Br Med J 1988; 297: 459–460.

Ray MJ, Padin DR, Condie JD et al. Charcoal bezoar. Small bowel obstruction secondary to amitriptyline overdose therapy. Dig Dis Sci 1988; 33: 106–107.

Whole bowel irrigation

Whole bowel irrigation is a newer method of gastric decontamination that is indicated for a limited number of poisons (see below). At present the evidence for whole bowel irrigation is based on case reports only. Whole bowel irrigation involves administration of non-absorbable polyethylene glycol solution to cause a liquid stool and reduce drug absorption by physically forcing gastrointestinal contents through the gut rapidly.

Indications for whole bowel irrigation:

- Large ingestions of agents not adsorbed to activated charcoal
  — iron
  — lithium
- Body packers, i.e. ingestion of drug-filled packets/condoms
- Large ingestions of sustained release or enteric coated drugs, e.g. theophylline.

Prior to the procedure check the patient does not have paralytic ileus. The procedure usually involves passing a nasogastric tube or persuading the patient to drink the polyethylene glycol. Commercially available polyethylene glycol preparations, often used in surgical units, are recommended such as Klean-Prep (60 g/L polyethylene glycol, with electrolytes). They are instilled at a rate of 2 L/hour in adults and

TABLE 1.9 Whole bowel irrigation complications and how to avoid them

Complication	Solution
Haemodynamic compromise	Do not use in patient with haemodynamic compromise from bleeding e.g. severe iron poisoning
Obstruction	Do not use in patients with ileus

0.5 L/hour in pre-school children. Watery diarrhoea soon develops and the patient is then sat on a commode. The polyethylene glycol is given until the rectal effluent becomes clear. Patients tolerate the procedure remarkably well. It even appears a safe procedure during pregnancy. Polyethylene glycol is not absorbed and does not result in changes in water or electrolyte balance.

> Warning! Polyethylene glycol is used. Do not use ethylene glycol – this is antifreeze and very toxic.

Further reading

American Academy of Clinical Toxicology; European Association of Poison Control Centres and Clinical Toxicologists. Position statement: Whole Bowel Irrigation. Clin Tox 1997; 35: 753–762.

Jones AL, Volans G. Management of self-poisoning. BMJ 1999; 319: 1414–1417.

Tenenbein M. Whole bowel irrigation as a gastrointestinal decontamination procedure after acute poisoning. Med Toxicol 1988; 3: 77–84.

Van Ameyde KJ, Tenenbein M. Whole bowel irrigation during pregnancy. Am J Obstet Gynecol 1989; 160: 646–647.

METHODS FOR ENHANCING ELIMINATION OF TOXINS

In the vast majority of patients who present after an overdose, gut decontamination methods and supportive care are all that is necessary. In a limited number of poisonings it may be necessary to consider the use of one of the methods that are available to increase elimination of poisons – these include urinary alkalinisation, multiple-dose activated charcoal and the extracorporeal techniques of haemodialysis, haemoperfusion and haemofiltration.

Multiple-dose activated charcoal

Repeated doses of activated charcoal can increase the elimination of some drugs by interrupting their entero-enteric and enterohepatic circulation. Clinical studies have shown that multiple-dose activated charcoal increases the elimination of certain drugs, but no controlled studies have established beyond doubt a clinical benefit on patient outcome, though this would seem logical.

The dose given is 50 g (1 g/kg in children) of activated charcoal every 4 hours.

Indications for multiple-dose activated charcoal include life-threatening overdose with:

- Carbamazepine
- Dapsone
- Phenobarbitone
- Quinine
- Theophylline.

Further reading
American Academy of Clinical Toxicologists; European Association of Poison Control Centres and Clinical Toxicologists. Position statement and practice guidelines on the use of multi-dose activated charcoal in the treatment of acute poisoning. Clin Tox 1999; 37(6): 731–751.

Urinary alkalinisation (also known as alkaline diuresis)
Indicated for serious poisoning with:

- Chlorpropamide
- Mecoprop
- Phenobarbitone
- Phenoxyacetate herbicides, e.g. 2,4-D
- Salicylates including aspirin.

Prior to the procedure check the patient's plasma potassium oncentration and renal function tests. Give intravenous bicarbonate 1 litre of 1.26% (for an adult) over 3 hours. Check plasma potassium, as it is very difficult to produce an alkaline urine if the patient is hypokalaemic. Also potassium can fall precipitously once adequate urinary alkalinisation commences and so it is wise to add 20–40 mmol potassium to each litre of i.v. fluids given. Check that adequate urinary alkalisation is achieved (aiming for a urinary pH of 7.5–8.5) by checking the pH of the urine with indicator paper.

> Warning! Never force a diuresis, as pulmonary oedema will ensue.
> Acetazolamide should never be used to induce an alkaline urine as it produces a systemic acidosis which enhances the toxicity of certain drugs such as salicylates.

Further reading
Prescott LF, Balali-Mood M, Critchley JAJH, Johnstone AF. Diuresis or urinary alkalinisation for salicylate poisoning? BMJ 1982; 285: 1383–1386.

Extracorporeal techniques: haemodialysis, charcoal haemoperfusion, haemofiltration
There are a limited number of poisonings in which one of these procedures may be indicated. Before deciding whether or not to undertake one of these procedures in a poisoned patient, the case should be discussed with a clinical toxicologist.

Patients undergoing these extracorporeal drug removal procedures will need to be in an intensive care/high dependency unit. Haemodialysis is only available in a limited number of centres in the UK. Charcoal haemoperfusion columns are not widely available. However if charcoal haemoperfusion is clinically indicated columns can be obtained from the manufacturer 24 hours a day and from some poisons centres. There is limited data on the use of haemofiltration in poisoned patients and at present we do not recommend its use.

TABLE 1.10   Indications for haemoperfusion and haemodialysis in poisoned patients

Drugs for which haemodialysis may be considered	Drugs for which charcoal haemoperfusion may be considered
Salicylates (see p. 80)	Theophylline (see p. 86)
Ethylene Glycol, Methanol, Ethanol (see pp. 110, 112)	Phenobarbitone
Theophylline (see p. 86)	Carbamazepine (see p. 42)
Lithium (see p. 60)	

TABLE 1.11   Extracorporeal technique complications and how to avoid them

Complication	Solution
Hypotension	Gradually increase flow rates in the extracorporeal circuit. Remember that hypotension may be due to the poisoning!
Air embolism	Carefully prime the extracorporeal circuit
Sepsis	Strict aseptic technique during central line insertion
Thrombocytopenia	Anticoagulation with prostacyclin rather than heparin
Bleeding	Careful monitoring of anticoagulation

For all of these procedures, central access with a double lumen catheter in a large vein (femoral, internal jugular or subclavian) is required. The extracorporeal circuit must be primed before use and anticoagulated – this is generally done with heparin, but prostacyclin may be used as an alternative, particularly in thrombocytopenic patients.

MANAGEMENT OF PATIENTS

Attitude

Self-poisoned patients do not always meet with the sympathies of the admitting medical team. Try to think of such patients as medical challenges rather than merely instances of self-inflicted illness. Care for such patients is a multidisciplinary responsibility and nurses, psychiatrists, physicians, occupational therapists and social workers all have key roles in the rehabilitation of the patient, as do friends and relatives. Take time to get to know the patient well. Give appropriate explanations and reassurance. Avoid unnecessarily large ward rounds and talking over the patient. Always explain procedures to the patient.

Admission policy
Admit:

- Anyone taking an overdose, however apparently trivial in amount.
- Anyone with self-harm, e.g. wrist slashing.

Threatened self-harm, however, is the responsibility of the duty psychiatrist rather than the admitting medical team.

Chemical exposures

Remove the patient from continued exposure to the chemical. If the toxin is a gas, the patient should be removed to fresh air or given supplemental high flow oxygen.

Avoid self-contamination: protective clothing (e.g. gloves, gowns, respiratory equipment) should be worn by medical and nursing staff. Decontamination should be carried out in a well-ventilated area. To minimise contamination the patient should remove contaminated clothing and wash him/herself if possible. Soiled clothing should be sealed in bags. The skin should be thoroughly washed with soap and water.

Eyes which have been exposed to acids, alkalis, chemicals or irritants should be thoroughly irrigated for at least 20 minutes with normal saline. They should then undergo slit-lamp examination with fluorescein drops. If any dye uptake indicative of corneal damage is seen, referral to an ophthalmologist is indicated.

> Warning! Thorough decontamination should ideally take place before a patient enters the accident and emergency department. Do not contaminate either yourself or your department.

Intubation and assisted ventilation

Indications for intubation and assisted ventilation:

- GCS <8 or falling rapidly.
- Recurrent seizures.
- Hypoxia – not corrected with oxygen mask and high flow oxygen.
- Hypercarbia (pCO_2 >6.6 kPa) or hypocarbia (pCO_2 <2.5 kPa).
- Inability to protect airway.
- Shock state, i.e. tachycardia, hypotension, metabolic acidosis.
- After a cardiac or respiratory arrest.

> Warning! Occasionally, a patient with a GCS >8 may require intubation if their airway is not maintained.

Optimising cardiac output and blood pressure

This encompasses maintenance of cardiac output and oxygen delivery as well as maintenance of adequate organ perfusion pressure or blood pressure (BP). Hypotension usually responds to adequate filling with i.v. fluids (see p. 17). The best approach to hypotension is to optimise fluid status, treat any cardiac arrhythmias and then add an inotrope or vasoconstrictor if required (see p. 17).

Fluids and electrolytes

Daily requirements of water are 30–35 ml/kg/day, Na^+ 1–1.5 mmol/kg/day, K^+ 1 mmol/kg/day. These requirements can be provided by 2–3 litres of fluid per day with additional potassium of 20 mmol/L. This will obviously be altered by factors such as renal failure, sepsis, burns, diarrhoea, hyperthermia or pre-existing dehydration. Colloids or crystalloid fluids should be used to treat hypotension. Albumin is not currently recommended for such use.

Inotropes and vasoconstrictors

Adrenaline increases heart rate and stroke volume. It is used at a dose of 0.1–0.5 µg/kg/min. At low doses, the primary effect is increased cardiac output, whilst at higher doses there is additional potent vasoconstriction. It is useful in low output states with low peripheral vasomotor tone and low mean arterial pressure (MABP). It is the drug of choice in emergency hypotensive states when the overall haemodynamic status is not clear.

> Warning! If a drug which sensitises the myocardium to the action of adrenaline has been taken, e.g. tricyclic antidepressants or amphetamines, use of adrenaline may precipitate arrhythmias.

Dobutamine increases heart rate and cardiac output but causes peripheral and splanchnic vasodilatation. It is used at a dose of 1–20 µg/kg/min. It is useful in low cardiac output states when the blood pressure is reasonably maintained.

At low doses (up to 5 µg/kg/min) the primary action of **dopamine** is on dopamine receptors and this increases splanchnic and renal perfusion. It may therefore be useful in helping to maintain renal blood flow and promote urine output, though it has unproven value in the treatment of renal failure. At doses above 5 µg/kg/min dopamine is a predominant vasoconstrictor and cardiac effects predominate.

If despite adequate filling and best achievable cardiac output, the MABP remains low, then vasoconstrictors should be used. Such agents include **noradrenaline** (0.1–0.5 µg/kg/min). Noradrenaline has no appreciable effect on cardiac output but it is useful in generating an adequate perfusion pressure for vital organs, in particular the brain, liver and kidneys. However, it should be used at the lowest possible dose to achieve the desired effect as it reduces renal blood flow, reduces splanchnic blood flow and impairs peripheral perfusion.

> Warning! Inotropes and vasoconstrictors are of little value if the circulation is empty.

Treating arrhythmias

Factors predisposing poisoned patients to arrhythmias include:

- Cardiotoxic drug ingestion
- Hypoxia
- Pain and anxiety
- Hypercarbia
- Electrolyte disturbance
- Hypovolaemia
- Underlying ischaemic heart disease.

Warning! In all cases of arrhythmias, give oxygen, check electrolytes and establish i.v. access. Try to avoid use of antiarrhythmic drugs, as they are all arrhythmogenic and you can get into a descending spiral of negative inotropic and chronotropic activity.

Sinus tachycardia often represents an appropriate response to a stimulus and is a common finding in overdose patients. Beta-blockers should not be given as decompensation may then occur. Most children and healthy adults will be able to tolerate a sinus tachycardia with a rate of up to 160–180 beats per min.

Sinus bradycardia. As the heart rate falls initially the cardiac output is maintained by an increase in stroke volume, but as the heart rate falls further the cardiac output and the BP will fall. Junctional or other escape rhythms may then appear. If bradycardia occurs, with significant hypotension, consider giving atropine 0.6 mg i.v. (up to a max of 3 g). If there is no satisfactory response to these measures, transvenous pacing or external pacing may be necessary – get help (p. 20)! An isoprenaline infusion can be used as a holding measure – start at 1 μg/kg/min and increase as necessary. Use the following specific antidotes if appropriate:

- Beta-blocker overdose – use glucagon (p. 39).
- Calcium antagonist overdose – use calcium gluconate or calcium chloride (p. 40).
- Digoxin overdose – use Fab fragments (p. 49).

Supraventricular tachycardia (SVT) includes all tachyarrhythmias originating above the ventricles. In SVT the QRS complexes are narrow, unless there is a conduction defect. Appropriate management depends on the degree of haemodynamic disturbance. If the patient is haemodynamically compromised with SVT consider sedation and synchronised cardioversion at 50 J, 100 J, 200 J and then 300 J. If the patient is more stable then adenosine 3 mg i.v. by bolus repeated if necessary every 1–2 minutes using 6 mg and then 12 mg can be used. Alternatively esmolol can be used (dose 40 mg i.v.

over 1 min + infusion of 4 mg/min up to a max of 12 mg/min). Overdrive pacing is a suitable alternative (p. 20).

Broad complex tachycardia should be assumed to be ventricular unless proven otherwise. Ventricular tachycardia is more likely if:

- The QRS on the ECG is very broad.
- There is evidence of AV dissociation (capture beats or fusion beats).
- There is a dominant first R wave in V1.
- There is a deep S wave in V6.
- The QRS direction is the same in all leads, i.e. concordance.

Management of broad complex tachycardia:

- With no cardiac output – DC cardioversion 200 J, 200 J, then 360 J, CPR and proceed as per standard European Resuscitation Council Guidelines.
- With output but with haemodynamic compromise – sedation and synchronised DC cardioversion 50 J, 100 J, then 200 J. If the patient has taken a tricyclic antidepressant drug overdose give 50–100 ml 8.4% sodium bicarbonate i.v. for an adult.
- With normal BP (unusual!) – treatment options depend on what the cause is. The general rule is to limit the use of antiarrhythmic agents – give oxygen and correct any electrolyte disturbances. If broad complex rhythm persists consider the use of prophylactic DC cardioversion or an agent such as lignocaine (100 mg i.v. bolus followed by infusion of 4 mg/min) for an adult, phenytoin 15 mg/kg i.v. over 20 mins for an adult or esmolol (i.v. 40 mg over 1 min followed by infusion of 4 mg/min up to a max of 12 mg/min) for an adult. If the patient has taken a tricyclic antidepressant give 50–100 ml 8.4% sodium bicarbonate i.v.

Torsade de pointes (polymorphic ventricular tachycardia) is like ventricular tachycardia except that the complexes vary from beat to beat with a constant change of axis. It may give rise to ventricular fibrillation. Common causes include hypokalaemia, drugs which prolong the QT interval and antiarrhythmic drugs. In the treatment of torsades, the following may be of value:

- 10 mmol magnesium sulphate i.v. (in children 0.08–0.16 mmol/kg) stat followed by 50 mmol infusion over 12 hours.
- Overdrive pacing (see p. 20).
- Cardioversion.
- Phenytoin 5 mg/kg i.v. over 20 minutes.

Ventricular fibrillation, asystole and **electromechanical dissociation** should all be treated according to standard European resuscitation guidelines.

Further reading
Advanced Life Support Working Group of the European Resuscitation Council 1998.

The European Resuscitation Council guidelines for adult advanced life support. BMJ 1998; 316: 1863–1869.

Transvenous pacing

This is often useful to overcome recurrent arrhythmias in patients who have taken cardiotoxic drugs. If recurrent VT is the main problem then overdrive pacing at or just above 120 bpm can protect against further arrhythmias. It is also very useful in bradycardia or heart block with haemodynamic compromise. However, do not pace a patient just to treat the bradycardia, if it is not causing hypotension. Often a higher pacing threshold (e.g. 1 volt) is required to achieve ventricular capture in a poisoned patient. Isoprenaline infusion can be used to 'hold' a patient until a person with pacing skills is available but in poisoned patients isoprenaline may precipitate arrhythmias, particularly where the myocardium is sensitised to endogenous catecholamines (p. 18).

> Warning! Paced patients in chest pain may be having ischaemia but you will not see it on the paced ECG – be vigilant.

Antidotes

Despite popular misconceptions, antidotes are available for only a small number of poisons:

TABLE 1.12 Antidotes	
Poison	*Antidote*
Anticoagulants	Vitamin K Fresh frozen plasma
Beta-blockers	Glucagon Adrenaline or Isoprenaline
Cyanide	Oxygen Dicobalt edetate Nitrites (inhaled amyl nitrite, i.v. sodium nitrite) Sodium thiosulphate Hydroxocobalamin
Ethylene glycol/Methanol	Ethanol 4-methylpyrazole
Lead	DMSA (2,3-dimercaptosuccinic acid) Disodium calcium edetate
Mercury	DMPS (2,3-dimercapto-1-propanesulphonate)
Iron salts	Desferrioxamine
	(Contd.)

TABLE 1.12 *(Continued)*	
Poison	*Antidote*
Opioids	Naloxone (Naltrexone)
Organophosphorus insecticides, nerve agents	Atropine Pralidoxime (P2S)
Paracetamol	N-acetylcysteine Methionine
Thallium	Prussian blue

Naloxone should be given as a 1.2–2 mg i.v. bolus for an adult, repeated as necessary. Infusion is often needed as the half-life of the antidote is much shorter than the half-life of most opioids (p. 67). The hourly infusion dose is two-thirds of the dose that was required as a bolus to wake up the patient.

Methaemoglobinaemia

Methaemoglobin (metHb) is an oxidised form of haemoglobin, which is incapable of carrying oxygen. Many oxidant drugs can cause methaemoglobinaemia (Table 1.13). The common agents are dapsone, nitrites, nitrates and local anaesthetics including lignocaine.

TABLE 1.13 **Agents capable of causing methaemoglobinaemia**	
Agent type	*Name*
Local anaesthetics	Benzocaine, lignocaine, prilocaine
Antibiotics	Dapsone, sulphonamides, trimethoprim
Nitrites and nitrates	Amyl nitrite, butyl nitrite, isobutyl nitrite, sodium nitrate, sodium nitrite
Others	Aniline dyes, bromates, chlorates, metoclopramide, methylene blue

Clinical Effects
The characteristic feature of methaemoglobinaemia is 'slate-grey' cyanosis. The severity of symptoms roughly correlates with measured methaemoglobin levels (Table 1.14). However, the figures given in the table assume normal total haemoglobin concentration – an anaemia will lead to more severe symptoms at a lower proportional methaemoglobin. Features will also be worse in patients with underlying medical disorders that may worsen hypoxaemia (e.g. pulmonary disease, heart failure).

TABLE 1.14   Clinical effects of methaemoglobin

Methaemoglobin concentration	Clinical effects
0–15%	None observed
15–30%	Mild effects; cyanosis, fatigue, dizziness, headache, nausea
30–50%	Moderate effects; marked cyanosis, weakness, tachypnoea, tachycardia, dyspnoea
50–70%	Severe effects; coma, convulsions, respiratory depression, arrhythmias, metabolic acidosis
>70%	Potentially fatal

The onset and duration of symptoms will depend on the agent causing methaemoglobinaemia. Nitrites cause symptoms within seconds or minutes of inhalation and they also cause vasodilation with flushing, headache and hypotension; the symptoms are usually moderate and short lived unless exposure is prolonged. In contrast ingestion of dapsone may be associated with a delay of onset of symptoms of several hours and methaemoglobinaemia can persist for several days. Dapsone can also cause sulphaemoglobinaemia and prolonged haemolysis.

Patients should have arterial blood gas and methaemoglobin concentration measured. Blood samples for methaemoglobin should be analysed as soon as possible because if left to stand the metHb concentration will be falsely low owing to reduction by endogenous methaemoglobin reductase. Blood should also be taken for FBC, particularly if dapsone has been taken.

Methaemoglobinaemia characteristically causes a normal pO_2 in the presence of decreased *measured* oxygen saturations. However, pulse oximetry will pick up both oxyHb and metHb and so will give falsely reassuring results.

Protect the airway, ventilate if necessary and give high flow oxygen. Contaminated clothing should be removed and exposed skin washed with soapy water. If dapsone has been ingested give multiple-dose activated charcoal (p. 13), ensuring that the airway is protected.

In patients with mild symptoms or methaemoglobin <30%, removal from the exposure and oxygen are usually the only treatment required. Dapsone can cause methaemoglobin formation and haemolysis for 2–3 days after ingestion and so prolonged observation may be necessary.

If the patient has severe clinical features (coma, convulsions, respiratory depression, hypotension, metabolic acidosis) or if the methaemoglobin level is >30% the patient should be given methylene blue.

Warning! Methylene blue may need to be given at lower methaemoglobin concentrations in those who are symptomatic.

The dose of methylene blue is 1–2 mg/kg body weight (0.1–0.2 ml/kg body weight of 1% solution) given over 5 minutes. The methaemoglobin concentration should be rechecked 1 hour after giving methylene blue and further doses of methylene blue may be required in severe cases. However, large doses of methylene blue (particularly > 15 mg/kg body weight) can cause methaemoglobinaemia itself and haemolysis, and so further doses should not be given unless clinically indicated.

Patients with glucose-6-phosphate dehydrogenase (G-6-PD) deficiency are very susceptible to methylene blue induced haemolysis. Also, methylene blue will be less effective in reducing methaemoglobin in G-6-PD deficiency. The treatment of methaemoglobinaemia in patients with G-6-PD deficiency should be discussed with a physician at a poisons centre.

Further reading
Hall AH, Kulig KW, Rumack BH. Drug and chemical induced methaemoglobinaemia. Clinical features and management. Med Toxicol 1986; 1: 232–260.

Griffin JP. Methaemoglobinaemia. Adv Drug React Toxicol 1997; 16(1): 45–63.

Persistent vomiting

If vomiting fails to respond to simple measures such as sucking ice cubes, metoclopramide 10 mg i.v. or orally, prochlorperazine 10 mg orally, or ondansetron may be particularly effective (8 mg by slow i.v. injection). Ondansetron seems to work particularly well in paracetamol or theophylline poisoning.

Dystonias

Dystonic reactions are common after overdoses with antipsychotic drugs and some anti-emetics. Dystonic reactions that can occur include oculo-gyric crises, torticollis (wry neck) and trismus (jaw clenching). Other extra-pyramidal features (tremor, dyskinesias, rigidity) may be seen with these and many other agents in overdose. Extrapyramidal symptoms should be treated with procyclidine (adults: 5–10 mg i.v. or i.m. to a maximum of 20 mg/24 hours; children: < 2 years 0.5–2 mg, > 2 years 2–5 mg, > 10 years 5–10 mg i.m. or i.v., repeated after 20 minutes if necessary) or benztropine (adults: 1–2 mg i.m. or i.v. repeated as required; children: 20 μg/kg/dose i.m., i.v. or p.o.). Further oral doses may be required for 24–48 hours to prevent recurrence of the dystonia.

Seizures or fits

These are a common complication of poisoning with a variety of drugs – see anticonvulsants (pp. 42, 77, 93), tricyclic antidepressants (p. 90), theophylline (p. 86) and NSAIDs (p. 65). A non-sustained fit does not require pharmacological intervention. However, persistent (lasting > 5 minutes) or recurrent seizures require treatment. The first line drug is i.v. diazepam (0.1–0.2 mg/kg body weight). This can be repeated two or three times as required. If seizures are persistent or recurrent despite adequate doses of benzodiazepines, phenytoin should be used (15 mg/kg at a rate not exceeding 50 mg per minute as a loading dose, followed by maintenance doses of about 100 mg for an adult given every 6–8 hours). In the worst case scenario, paralysis and ventilation may be necessary, with EEG monitoring to exclude ongoing seizure activity.

Sedation

Before sedating a patient, exclude possible causes of agitation such as hypoglycaemia, full bladder, pain, hypoxia and CO_2 retention. Sedation should be carried out with a benzodiazepine such as diazepam 5–10 mg i.v. bolus, or orally if the patient can be persuaded to take it, and repeated as necessary.

If benzodiazepines fail to control the patient, chlorpromazine (5–10 mg i.v. bolus in an adult) repeated as necessary, or haloperidol (5–10 mg i.v. in an adult) repeated as necessary can be used. Chlorpromazine and haloperidol are major tranquillisers, and they calm the patient without undue sedation or respiratory depression; however, they lower seizure threshold and so should be used with care if the patient has taken a drug that may cause seizures (see p. 23). They are of particular use in acute confusional states or when other agents are not working. Beware of hypotension due to alpha blockade and also beware of use in serotonergic states or hyperpyrexia (e.g. ecstasy intoxication), as they may make muscular rigidity and hyperpyrexia worse.

The following measures are advised when confronted with an aggressive or violent patient:

- Talk to the patient calmly, giving reassurance
- Avoid excessive eye contact
- Attempt to address the patient's immediate needs
- Maintain a buffer of at least two arm lengths
- Consider restraint
- Consider drug treatment (see above).

Rhabdomyolysis

Rhabdomyolysis may occur after drug overdose for a number of reasons:

- Pressure effect – prolonged unconsciousness with immobilisation in one position on a hard surface.
- Repeated seizures and/or hyperthermia (e.g. amphetamines, cocaine, strychnine).
- Rarely, due to a direct toxic effect of the drug (e.g. colchicine).

Rhabdomyolysis results in a raised serum creatinine kinase (CK) and myoglobinuria. Myoglobin can precipitate in the kidneys, particularly if the patient is dehydrated, leading to acute tubular necrosis and renal failure.

Patients with rhabdomyolysis should be kept well hydrated with intravenous fluids. For massive rhabdomyolysis (CK > 10 000 IU/L) urinary alkalinisation (p. 14) may be considered.

Anticholinergic syndrome

This occurs when a drug with prominent anticholinergic activity has been taken in overdose, such as tricyclic antidepressants (p. 90) and H_1-antihistamines (p. 33). The features include tachycardia, dilated pupils, hot dry skin and agitated delirium. There may be a twilight zone during improvement, when a patient stares vacantly into space and plucks at the bedclothes. There was once a fashion for treating such patients with physostigmine – this practice is both dangerous and ineffective. This is best treated by symptomatic and supportive care alone.

Neuroleptic malignant syndrome

This may be caused by any antipsychotic drug (e.g. chlorpromazine) as an adverse event at therapeutic doses or in overdoses. It is characterised by confusion, fluctuating consciousness, rigidity, tremor, autonomic instability, sweating, hyperpyrexia and rhabdomyolysis. It should be treated by withdrawal of the offending drug and maintenance of fluid and electrolyte balance. In severe cases, sedation with diazepam (0.1–0.2 mg/kg i.v. or orally) and application of cooling measures such as i.v. fluids and dantrolene (1 mg/kg i.v. over 15 minutes to a maximum of 10 mg/kg over a 24-hour period). In patients not responding to these measures, bromocriptine can be considered (2.5–10 mg 8-hourly, orally or through nasogastric tube).

Serotonin syndrome

This may be caused by interaction between MAOIs and many drugs including serotonin re-uptake inhibitors, dextromorphan and tricyclic antidepressants. It is characterised by agitation, tremor, clonus, hyperreflexia, hypertonia, sweating, tachycardia and hyperpyrexia. It should be treated by withdrawal of the offending drug and, if necessary in severe cases, sedation with diazepam and application of cooling measures (p. 52). In the future specific serotonergic agents may be used in patients with serotonin syndrome, e.g. chlorpromazine, cyproheptadine or ketanserin, to reduce temperature and rigidity by central mechanisms.

Management of bodypackers

Bodypackers are individuals who ingest drugs of abuse (particularly cocaine and heroin) wrapped in clingfilm or filled in condoms or the fingers of rubber gloves for the purpose of smuggling. Rupture of the packets can potentially be fatal because large doses are often put into the packets. If rupture does occur patients can deteriorate very rapidly.

 If bodypacking is suspected it is important to ascertain exactly what is in the packets as drugs such as cocaine or opioids are often high grade and leakage of even a small amount can cause death. Next it is important to X-ray the patient and see where the packets are located and how many are present. If they are in the stomach they can be removed endoscopically (taking extreme care not to rupture the packages) or allowed to pass thorough 'naturally' with the help of laxatives. Paraffin based laxatives should *not* be used as this may increase the risk of packet rupture.

> Warning! Gastric lavage should not be used as it may precipitate package rupture. If there are signs of rupture, e.g. cocaine or opioid toxicity, then urgent surgical removal of the packets is indicated.

If packages are in the small bowel or large bowel they can either be allowed to pass 'naturally' with laxatives or whole bowel irrigation can be performed to aid their speedy recovery (p. 12). Patients should be admitted and observed closely.

Packets 'stuffed' into the vagina or rectum can be removed manually.

Transporting poisoned patients

Sometimes seriously poisoned or potentially seriously poisoned patients may need to be moved to other hospitals or hyperbaric facilities. It is critically important that whoever takes the decision to move such patients weighs up the risk of transfer versus remaining at the original hospital – ideally this should be a consultant. If transport is arranged, it should always be with a medical escort who is competent at endotracheal intubation and treatment of cardiac arrhythmias. Resuscitation equipment, oxygen, suction equipment, together with a limited number of drugs such as adrenaline, calcium gluconate, lignocaine, benzodiazepines and oxygen should be carried. Ideally an ECG monitor and oxygen saturation monitor should be available throughout the transit, and this is *essential* if cardiotoxic drugs have been taken.

Prediction of outcome in poisoning

Difficulties in caring for poisoned patients and unexpected deaths have led to the development of scoring systems to predict risk. This generally involves the collection of a large amount of data to calculate a risk score for the patient. A number of scoring systems have been devised including the Poisons Severity Score (PSS) developed by the WHO. In some types of poisoning, outcome can be predicted by knowledge of the plasma concentration and time since overdose, e.g. paracetamol (p. 69) and paraquat poisoning (p. 120).

Further reading
Persson HE, Sjoberg GK, Haines JA, Pronczuk de Garbino J. Poisoning severity score. Grading of acute poisoning. Clin Tox 1998; 36: 205–213.

Talking to relatives

It is always wise to keep families abreast of what is happening to the patient. Discussions with relatives should generally take place in a quiet room away from the patient's beside.

Medico-legal issues

Patients who refuse treatment can present problems and the situation needs to be handled carefully. A mentally competent adult has every right to withhold consent to examination, investigation or medical treatment, even if such a decision may result in his or her death. It is therefore important that you are able to assess capacity for competence. It is often best that a third person, such as a nurse, witnesses such assessment and it is vital that adequate documentation is made.

Assessing capacity for competence: to show that they are competent to refuse medical treatment, patients

1. Must be able to understand and retain information on the treatment proposed – its indications, its main benefits, as well as possible risks and the consequences of non-treatment
2. Must be shown to believe that information
3. Must be capable of weighing up the information in order to arrive at a conclusion.

If a patient is capable of all three of these elements, refusal of treatment must be judged as valid and respected. However, it is essential to maintain a supportive approach, and the support of family and friends can be invaluable at this stage. An apparently irrational decision in itself does not compromise capacity – it is the process by which the patient arrives at the decision that is important. If there is any doubt on the assessment of capacity, get a second opinion, ideally from a psychiatrist.

A particularly difficult situation arises if a patient who has capacity but refuses treatment later becomes unconscious – in such circumstances treatment cannot be given in the absence of prior consent.

Treatment can only be given to a patient against their will in the following circumstances:

- If the patient is detainable under the Mental Health Act 1983. However, the Mental Health Act allows for treatment for mental disorders to be given without the patient's consent, but does *not* allow for medical treatment to be given without the patient's consent.
- Under common law if a patient lacks mental capacity, a doctor may administer any medical treatment essential to preserve life and considered to be in the patient's best interests. This also applies to the patient who is brought to the hospital unconscious requiring emergency treatment.

Children

In patients under the age of 16, assessment of the individual child's understanding will determine whether he or she can give consent to medical treatment – this is known as the assessment of Gillick competence. Consent by a competent child cannot be overridden by parental refusal, but the reverse fortunately does not apply. Children over 16 are treated as adults.

> Warning! Always document patient refusal to treatment carefully in the notes. Witnesses should be named and sign the records.
> Always seek help regarding more difficult ethical and legal decisions.
> Most patients can be persuaded to have treatment with a little charm and patience.

Further reading

Managing self-harm: the legal issues. Drugs and Therapeutics Bulletin 1997; 35(6): 41–43.

Hassan TB, MacNamara AF, Davy A, Bing A, Bodiwala GG. Managing patients with deliberate self-harm who refuse treatment in the accident and emergency department. BMJ 1999; 319: 107–109.

When are patients fit to be discharged?

In simplistic terms, patients are fit for discharge from inpatient care when they no longer require the specialist skills and monitoring available on the ward. This generally means they are alert, awake and orientated, have no life-threatening organ failure and have been passed psychiatrically safe for discharge. A psychiatric liaison nurse or doctor should assess *all* patients who have taken an overdose prior to discharge.

Where the patient will be sent will depend on a variety of factors, but most importantly the patient's mental state. Some patients, especially if family support is good, may be fit enough to return home after an overdose. Others may require psychiatric observation and nursing care.

Whenever a patient is transferred out of hospital, you must inform the general practitioner and usually also the community psychiatric nurse. You should provide a short written summary of what has been taken and what complications have occurred, together with a guide for on-going care and monitoring for professionals involved in further care.

Death

Once death is confirmed you must make sure the relatives have been informed. It is also important to inform the consultant and general practitioner. Where death by poisoning or suspected poisoning, self-harm or misuse of drugs has occurred, the death must be reported to a coroner (Procurator Fiscal in Scotland).

When speaking to the coroner's office you will need the following information:

- Deceased's name, date of birth, address
- Address and telephone number of next of kin and general practitioner
- Brief summary of last illness, including date of admission, suspected toxin, analytical confirmation, complications and time of death.

DRUGS AND DRUGS OF ABUSE

ACE INHIBITORS

Overdoses with ACE inhibitors such as enalapril, captopril or lisinopril cause remarkably few symptoms and signs. Features of toxicity include hypotension and reflex tachycardia. Hyperkalaemia and renal failure are uncommon. Hypotension should be treated with elevation of the foot of the bed and i.v. fluids. Inotropic agents are rarely necessary.

AMPHETAMINES: see ECSTASY

ANTIDIABETIC AGENTS – INSULIN, METFORMIN, SULPHONYLUREAS

These include the sulphonylureas (e.g. chlorpropamide, glibenclamide, gliclazide, glipizide, tolbutamide), biguanides (metformin) and insulin.

SULPHONYLUREAS AND INSULIN

These agents cause hypoglycaemia when taken in overdose (insulin is toxic if injected, but non-toxic if ingested orally). The onset and duration of hypoglycaemia varies according to the agent, but it can last for several days with longer acting drugs such as chlorpropamide and insulatard. Hypoglycaemia may manifest as agitation, sweating, confusion, tachycardia, hypotension, drowsiness, coma or convulsions. Permanent neurological effects can occur if hypoglycaemia is prolonged.

Activated charcoal should be given (and gastric lavage considered) to all patients who present within 1 hour of ingestion of more than the normal therapeutic dose of sulphonylureas. Formal blood glucose (not just BM) and U&Es should be checked and repeated regularly. Correct hypoglycaemia urgently with 50 ml 50% dextrose i.v. (1–2 ml/kg 50% dextrose for children) if the patient is unconscious, or a sugary drink if the patient is conscious.

This should be followed by an infusion of 10% or 20% dextrose given at a rate to prevent further hypoglycaemia, titrated against blood glucose/BMs. Potassium replacement is necessary and should be guided by frequent measurement of U&Es (as a general rule, add 10–20 mmol potassium chloride to each litre of dextrose). Octreotide should be considered after sulphonylurea overdose associated with prolonged hypoglycaemia. Patients may need dextrose infusions for several days depending on the agent ingested/injected. Failure to regain consciousness within a few minutes of normalisation of the blood glucose can indicate that a CNS depressant has also been ingested or that the patient has cerebral oedema. Cerebral oedema should be treated conventionally. Patients should be observed with hourly BMs for a minimum of 24 hours.

> Warning! It is desirable, but not essential to confirm hypoglycaemia before treatment – if in doubt treat.
> Beware of hypoglycaemia occurring 6–8 hours after the overdose, once liver glycogen is deplete.

METFORMIN

Metformin can cause a type-B lactic acidosis in overdose, particularly when it is co-ingested with ethanol, in elderly patients and in patients with renal or hepatic impairment. Clinical effects seen in overdose include nausea and vomiting, diarrhoea, abdominal pain and a severe lactic acidosis, which can result in hyperventilation, drowsiness, coma, hypotension and cardiovascular collapse. Hypoglycaemia can occur but is much less common than with sulphonylureas. Lactic acidosis associated with metformin is associated with a high (>50%) mortality. All patients should have blood taken for U&Es and venous bicarbonate. Arterial blood gases should be checked in symptomatic patients and those with a low plasma bicarbonate concentration (e.g. less than 20 mmol/L).

Activated charcoal should be given (and gastric lavage considered) in all patients who present within 1 hour of ingestion of a significant quantity of metformin. Metabolic acidosis should be treated with i.v. 1–2 ml/kg of 8.4% sodium bicarbonate repeated as necessary. Patients with a resistant metabolic acidosis should receive haemodialysis, which as well as correcting the metabolic acidosis will also clear metformin.

(H₁) ANTIHISTAMINES

H₁ antihistamines are commonly found in over-the-counter and prescription medications used for hay fever, allergies, motion sickness, sleep aids, and cough and cold preparations. The older sedating antihistamines (e.g. azatadine, brompheniramine, chlorpheniramine, clemastine, cyproheptadine, diphenhydramine, doxylamine, hydroxyzine, phenindamine, pheniramine, promethazine, trimeprazine) have anticholinergic effects in overdose, the newer non-sedating ones (e.g. astemizole, cetirizine, fexofenadine, loratadine, terfenadine) produce few or no anticholinergic effects. Astemizole and terfenadine can cause QT_c prolongation and torsade de pointes (p. 19), this can occur after an overdose or after use of an interacting drug (e.g. erythromycin, ketoconazole).

Clinical features

Clinical effects in overdose include drowsiness and/or agitation, nausea and vomiting and anticholinergic effects (dilated pupils, tachycardia, dry mouth, delirium, hallucinations, pyrexia). In severe cases, convulsions, rhabdomyolysis and hypotension can occur. Coma is rare. Massive diphenhydramine overdose has been reported to cause QRS widening and ventricular arrhythmias similar to those from tricyclic antidepressants. The newer non-sedating antihistamines tend to cause fewer effects in overdose with the exception of terfenadine and astemizole, which can cause prolongation of the QT_c and ventricular arrhythmias, particularly torsade de pointes (p. 19).

Activated charcoal should be given within 1 hour of ingestion for all but trivial overdoses. An ECG should be carried out on all symptomatic patients and all patients who have taken astemizole or terfenadine. Patients should be observed with ECG monitoring for at least 8 hours after overdose (12 hours for slow release preparations). Patients who have taken terfenadine or astemizole should be observed with ECG monitoring for at least 12 hours after overdose and until the QT_c has returned to normal. The treatment of choice for arrhythmias associated with terfenadine and astemizole is i.v. magnesium (10 mmol as a bolus followed by 50 mmol infusion over 12 hours for an adult) together with overdrive pacing (p. 20) or DC cardioversion.

BACLOFEN

Baclofen is used to treat skeletal muscle spasticity, particularly in multiple sclerosis. Overdose of greater than 100 mg will usually produce symptoms and greater than 150 mg can be associated with severe toxicity in an adult. Onset of symptoms is rapid and effects can last for up to 35–40 hours. Features include drowsiness, coma, respiratory depression, hypotonia, hyporeflexia, hypothermia and hypotension. Bradycardia with first-degree AV block and QT_c prolongation can occur. During recovery, agitation, convulsions and myoclonic jerks can occur.

Management is supportive and often requires intensive care. Activated charcoal should be given (and gastric lavage should be considered) for ingestion of >100 mg by an adult (1.4 mg/kg in a child) presenting within 1 hour. Convulsions should be treated with i.v. diazepam 0.1–0.2 mg/kg.

BENZODIAZEPINES

In general benzodiazepine overdoses are remarkably safe and almost full recovery takes place within 24 hours. However, performance in skilled tasks may be impaired for several days after apparent recovery and patients should be warned not to drive or operate machinery.

Difficulties in benzodiazepine overdosage occur when they are mixed with other CNS depressant sedatives such as tricyclic antidepressants, opioids or alcohol, or when the elderly or those with chronic obstructive pulmonary disease take them.

Common benzodiazepines involved in overdose:

- Chlordiazepoxide
- Clonazepam
- Diazepam
- Flunitrazepam
- Lometazepam
- Lorazepam
- Lorazolam
- Midazolam
- Nitrazepam
- Temazepam.

Zopiclone is a benzodiazepine-like sedative that behaves similarly in overdose to benzodiazepines.

Clinical features

Drowsiness and mid-position or dilated pupils are common and commonly occur within 3 hours of ingestion. Ataxia, dysarthria and nystagmus, and confusion or agitation can occur. Coma may follow, but in lone benzodiazepine overdose this is seldom less than GCS grade 10 and usually lasts less than 24 hours. Minor systemic hypotension and respiratory depression may occur. Bradycardia has been reported but is usually not clinically significant. Patients with benzodiazepine coma tend to be hyporeflexic. Respiratory arrest is uncommon but more likely after shorter acting agents such as triazolam or midazolam.

> Warning! Beware of mixed overdoses.
> Don't use flumazenil in the vast majority of cases. Flumazenil must *not* be used in patients with a history of convulsions, toxin-induced cardiotoxicity, or those who have co-ingested tricyclic antidepressants.

Essential laboratory investigations
None.

Supportive care

Gastric lavage is not advised in pure benzodiazepine overdose. Activated charcoal can be given within 1 hour of the overdose, but is superfluous in the context of quite low toxicity. Multiple-dose activated charcoal is not indicated.

Impairment of consciousness should be treated conventionally, with particular attention to maintenance of the airway. Observation should be for at least 6 hours post-ingestion, or for 24 hours in more serious cases if the patient is still symptomatic at 6 hours post-ingestion. Pulse oximetry is useful for monitoring adequacy of ventilation if significant CNS depression is present.

Specific measures

Flumazenil is a specific benzodiazepine antagonist but it is not used in the vast majority of cases of poisoning with benzodiazepines. It is not licensed for such use by the CSM in the UK. Flumazenil *must never be* used in patients with a history of convulsions, toxin-induced cardiotoxicity or those who have co-ingested tricyclic antidepressants. If given to such patients, seizures and ventricular arrhythmias can be precipitated. It may precipitate acute withdrawal (including seizures) in patients who are addicted to benzodiazepines.

Its use could be *considered* after the above contraindications have been excluded in patients with deep coma (e.g. GCS < 8) in doses of 500 µg i.v. in adults, repeated at 1-minute intervals until the patient wakes or to a maximum dose of 3 mg. It may be followed by infusion at 0.5–1 mg/hour for an adult, if there is response, to maintain the response, as the half-life of flumazenil is shorter than benzodiazepines and their metabolites. Complications of flumazenil use include convulsions, bradycardia, VT and complete heart block. The risk of these complications is reduced by using titrated doses as above and by excluding high risk patients such as those listed above.

There is no role for haemodialysis or charcoal haemoperfusion in benzodiazepine overdose.

Further reading

Haverkos GP, DiSalvo RP, Imhoff TE. Fatal seizures after flumazenil administration in a patient with a mixed drug overdose. Ann Pharmacother 1994; 28: 1347–1349.

Herd B, Clarke F. Complete heart block after flumazenil. Hum Exp Tox 1991; 10: 289.

Geller E, Crome P, Schaller MD, Marchant B, Ectors M, Scollo-Lavizzari G. Risks and benefits of therapy with flumazenil (Anexate) in mixed drug intoxications. Eur Neurol 1991; 31: 241–250.

Haverkos GP, DiSalvo RP, Imhoff TE. Fatal seizures after flumazenil administration in a patient with mixed overdose. Ann Pharmacotherapy 1994; 28: 1347–1349.

McDuffee AT, Tobias JD. Seizure after flumazenil administration in a paediatric patient. Pediatr Emerg Care 1995; 11: 186–187.

BETA-BLOCKERS

Beta-blockers are widely used antihypertensive and anti-anginal agents. They are also used to treat arrhythmias, anxiety, glaucoma, thyrotoxicosis, and as migraine prophylaxis. Some beta-blockers, e.g. atenolol and bisoprolol, are more 'cardioselective' (see Table 2.1) than others, i.e. they more selectively block β_1 receptors rather than β_2 receptors at therapeutic doses, resulting in fewer side effects. This selectivity decreases with increasing dose of the beta-blocker, and is usually irrelevant in overdose. Some beta-blockers, such as pindolol, have partial agonist activity, i.e. they may partially stimulate β_1 receptors – in overdose these drugs may cause tachycardia and hypertension. Lipophilic beta-blockers are more likely to cross into the brain, and consequently cause central nervous system effects. For example, propranolol is lipophilic and causes a number of CNS effects in overdose, such as delirium, hallucinations and seizures, even in the absence of hypotension. Atenolol is not lipophilic, and has fewer effects on the CNS in overdose. Some beta-blockers, such as propanolol, have membrane-stabilising effects (see Table 2.1). These agents are more likely to cause myocardial depression and rhythm disturbances in overdose.

TABLE 2.1   Properties of beta-blockers

Drug	Cardioselectivity	Membrane stabilisation	Partial agonist activity	Other
Acebutolol	+	+	+	
Atenolol	+	0	0	
Bisoprolol	+	0	0	
Esmolol	+	0	0	
Labetolol	0	+	0	Alpha-blocking activity
Metoprolol	+	+/−	0	
Pindolol	0	+	+ + +	
Propanolol	0	+ +	0	
Sotalol	0	0	0	Class III antiarrhythmic activity

Clinical features

Individual response to beta-blocker overdose is variable, and those with cardiac disease are at more risk of toxicity, particularly of complications such as pulmonary oedema. Patients on chronic beta-blocker therapy may have some resistance to the effects of overdose. Ingestion of other antihypertensive agents will potentiate the toxicity of beta-blockers, and may complicate treatment of the overdose. Agents that are particularly of concern include diltiazem and verapamil. Toxicity from beta-blockers can persist even after the drug is no longer detectable in the blood.

> Warning! Care should be taken to identify whether or not the preparation is sustained release if propranolol, metoprolol or oxprenolol have been ingested. Toxicity can be delayed and prolonged with these preparations.

Effects may appear quickly after ingestion, especially with substantial overdoses. For standard release preparations, effects are most commonly reported to begin within 2 hours of ingestion, and most patients who will be symptomatic develop effects within 4 hours of ingestion. Hypotension and bradycardia are common. Overdose with beta-blockers possessing partial agonist activity may lead to tachycardia and hypertension. Other cardiac effects include prolonged PR interval, first-degree AV block and bundle branch block. Severe toxicity may result in disappearance of P waves, prolongation of the QRS interval or QT interval (e.g. sotalol), complete heart block, asystole and ventricular fibrillation. Cardiogenic shock and pulmonary oedema can occur, especially in patients with pre-existing cardiac disease.

CNS effects such as drowsiness, dilated pupils, hallucinations, coma, convulsions and respiratory depression are more commonly seen in overdose with beta-blockers that are able to penetrate the CNS or have membrane stabilising activity.

> Warning! Bronchospasm may occur in susceptible individuals, such as asthmatics or those with chronic obstructive pulmonary disease.

Essential investigations
An ECG is essential. Where bronchospasm is present, peak flow must be estimated. Hypoglycaemia has been reported, most often in diabetics and in children, and therefore frequent blood sugar estimations are advised in such groups. Blood levels of beta-blockers do not correlate well with toxicity, and measurement of levels is not relevant in the management of beta-blocker overdose.

Supportive care
For overdose of **non-sustained-release** formulations, activated charcoal is recommended (adult 50 g, child 1 g/kg) within 1 hour of the overdose and prior gastric lavage should also be considered in potentially life-threatening overdoses (p. 9). Atropine (adult: 0.6 mg; child: 0.03 mg/kg s.c. or i.v.) should be given prior to this procedure to prevent cardiovascular collapse, which may occur during gastric lavage in beta-blocked patients owing to unopposed vagal stimulation. Atropine should not be used if beta-blockers are co-ingested with drugs with anticholinergic properties (e.g. tricyclic antidepressants, antihistamines, phenothiazines). Observation with ECG monitoring for at least 6 hours is recommended, except for sotalol ingestions where observation should be for a minimum of 8 hours if asymptomatic and at least 24 hours if symptomatic. Monitor the heart rate, blood pressure, ECG, respiratory rate, and oxygen saturations. Have a low threshold for administration of supplemental oxygen. Treat convulsions with i.v. diazepam (0.1–0.2 mg/kg body weight). Nebulised beta-2-agonists such as salbutamol and terbutaline should be used to treat severe bronchospasm. Mechanical ventilation may be required for significant respiratory depression.

For overdose of **sustained-release** preparations, repeat-doses of activated charcoal (p. 13) and/or whole bowel irrigation (p. 12) should be considered. Although studies evaluating efficacy are lacking, there is a theoretical basis for their efficacy. Patients who have ingested sustained-release preparations should be observed with ECG monitoring until at least 12 hours post-ingestion.

Specific measures
The value of atropine for the routine treatment of beta-blocker-induced bradycardia is questionable. However, it should be used in patients with a bradycardia associated with hypotension (up to 3 mg i.v. for an adult,

0.4 mg/kg for a child). Hypotension should initially be treated with i.v. fluids; this should be done cautiously in patients with pre-existing cardiac disease or those at risk of serious poisoning. In such cases CVP (central venous pressure) monitoring is advisable.

Glucagon is the drug of choice for patients who are haemodynamically compromised. Adults should receive a 10 mg i.v. bolus, repeated as required or followed by an i.v. infusion at 1–10 mg/hr depending on response. Children can be given 50–150 µg/kg i.v. or up to 50 µg/kg/hr by i.v. infusion. Vomiting is a useful indicator that an adequate dose has been given. Occasionally an anti-emetic is required. Some patients do not respond to glucagon and if vomiting has occurred without an effect on the blood pressure, further glucagon is unlikely to be of benefit. Glucagon administration at these relatively large doses may also cause hyperglycaemia, so the blood glucose concentration must be monitored. Glucagon comes as a dried powder and should be dissolved in 5% dextrose (the diluent in the drug-pack should not be used when giving large doses because it contains phenol).

Adrenaline may be used when glucagon is ineffective. Adults and children should be given 1–5 µg/kg/min, titrating the dose to the response (p. 17). **Isoprenaline** could be tried if other therapies are unsuccessful – start at 1 µg/min and increase as necessary, titrating the dose to the response. Isoprenaline has the disadvantage that it may reduce the diastolic blood pressure owing to vasodilation, especially following ingestion of cardioselective beta-blockers. It is pro-arrhythmic and should be avoided following sotalol ingestion. **Cardiac pacing** should be considered if there is no response to drug therapy. However, the heart may be refractory to normal pacing potentials, which may need to be increased to higher levels before capture occurs (e.g. 1 volt) (p. 20). **Prolonged external cardiac massage** may be required in patients unresponsive to drug therapy or pacing.

In the treatment of **sotalol-induced ventricular arrhythmias** drug therapy should be avoided if possible. Use of class Ia (quinine, quinidine, procainamide, disopyramide) and class III (amiodarone) antiarrhythmics is contraindicated. Lignocaine is also contraindicated as it further reduces the blood pressure. Ventricular fibrillation should be treated conventionally according to European Resuscitation guidelines (p. 19). VT and torsade de pointes in an unconscious patient: synchronised DC cardioversion. VT and torsade de pointes in a conscious patient: an infusion of magnesium sulphate is recommended – the dose in adults is 10 mmol, repeated if necessary, in children 0.08–0.16 mmol/kg by slow i.v. injection. For persistent or recurrent VT or torsade de pointes overdrive pacing is the treatment of choice (p. 20).

Further reading

Lip GYH, Ferner RE. Poisoning with anti-hypertensive drugs: beta-adrenoceptor blocker drugs. J Hum Hypertension 1995; 9: 213–221.

Love JN. Beta blocker toxicity after overdose: when do symptoms develop in adults? J Emerg Med 1994; 12: 799–802.

Neuvonen PJ et al. Prolonged Q-T interval and severe tachyarrhythmias, common features of sotalol intoxication. Eur J Clin Pharmacology 1991; 20: 85–89.

Taboulet P et al. Pathophysiology and management of self poisoning with beta-blockers. Clin Toxicol 1993; 31: 531–551.

CALCIUM CHANNEL BLOCKERS

These include verapamil, diltiazem and the dihydropyridines (e.g. nifedipine, amlodipine, nimodipine) and are used for treatment of angina, hypertension and arrhythmias.

> Warning! Many of the agents are available in sustained-release preparations, which can result in delayed onset and sustained toxicity.

Overdose with calcium antagonists can result in life-threatening features and the toxic-therapeutic ratio is small, so severe effects can occur after any dose greater than the usual therapeutic range.

Clinical effects
The features of overdose usually appear within 2–4 hours, although they can be delayed for up to 18–24 hours if a sustained-release preparation has been taken. Cardiac effects dominate the clinical picture, particularly hypotension and bradycardia/AV block. Reflex tachycardia may occur with nifedipine. Hypotension is due to a combination of peripheral vasodilation, bradyarrhythmias and a negative inotropic effect. Other effects include nausea and vomiting, drowsiness and confusion, hyperglycaemia, hypokalaemia or hyperkalaemia, coma and, rarely, convulsions may occur.

Supportive care
Gastric lavage should be considered and activated charcoal given if a patient presents within 1 hour of a large overdose. The use of multiple-dose activated charcoal or whole bowel irrigation following overdose of sustained-release calcium channel blockers has not been evaluated, although there is a theoretical basis for their efficacy. Patients who have ingested a standard release preparation should be observed (with ECG monitoring) for at least 6–8 hours after overdose; observation after a sustained-release preparation should be for at least 18–24 hours. Use i.v. fluids cautiously in patients with hypotension, particularly if there is pre-existent cardiac disease, because of the risk of precipitating pulmonary oedema.

Specific management
Calcium salts have a beneficial effect in some patients (they may increase blood pressure, but rarely affect bradycardia). Calcium gluconate should be

given i.v. at a dose of 10–20 ml of 10% in an adult, repeated as necessary every 5–15 minutes (children 0.5 ml/kg of 10% calcium gluconate). Following administration of repeated doses of calcium it is necessary to check for hypercalcaemia. Glucagon (p. 39) may be used in patients with hypotension who do not respond to calcium salts. The i.v. dose is 10 mg for an adult, 50–150 µg/kg in a child. This can be repeated if a response is achieved. Inotropic drugs (p. 17) are frequently required in patients with resistant hypotension.

Atropine (0.6–1.2 mg i.v. for an adult, 0.02 mg/kg i.v. for a child) should be used for bradycardia with haemodynamic compromise. However, in unresponsive cases with profound bradycardia or heart block, transvenous pacing may be necessary (p. 20). Haemodialysis and haemoperfusion are ineffective.

Further reading

Lip GYH, Ferner RE. Poisoning with anti-hypertensive drugs: calcium antagonists. J Human Hypertension 1995; 9: 155–161.

Howarth DM, Dawson AH, Smith AJ, Buckley NA, Whyte IM. Calcium channel blocking drug overdose: an Australian series. Human Exp Toxicol 1994; 13: 161–166.

CANNABIS

Cannabis is the collective term for all psychoactive substances from the dried leaves and flowers of the plant *Cannabis sativa*. Marijuana refers to any part of the plant used to induce effects and hashish is the dried resin from the flower tops. Cannabis is usually dried and either smoked or eaten. Slang terms include hash, grass, pot, ganja, spliff and reefer.

Clinical features

The clinical effects experienced by a particular individual depend on their mood, personality, environment and the dose taken.

After smoking, the onset of effects is 10–30 minutes, after ingestion the onset is 1–3 hours. The duration of effects is 4–8 hours. Low doses of cannabis produce euphoria, perceptual alterations, followed by relaxation and drowsiness. Hypertension, tachycardia, slurred speech, ataxia and appetite stimulation may also occur. High doses produce acute paranoid psychosis, anxiety, depersonalisation, confusion, hallucinations and distortion of time and space.

Ataxia, nystagmus, dilated pupils, tremor, stupor, conjunctival hyperaemia, tachycardia and confusion have been reported in children after ingestion of cannabis. These effects resolve in 6–12 hours.

Intravenous abuse of the crude extract of cannabis may cause nausea and vomiting, diarrhoea, abdominal pain, fever, hypotension, pulmonary oedema, acute renal failure, disseminated intravascular coagulation and death.

Essential investigations

Most patients have only mild symptoms after cannabis exposure and so unless severe systemic effects are present no investigations are needed.

Cannabinoid metabolites may be detected in the urine for several days after acute exposure, but urine levels do not correlate with the degree of toxicity.

Supportive care

Activated charcoal should be given for any amount of cannabis ingested by a child within an hour. This should be followed by observation for a minimum of 6 hours.

Serious cases from ingestion or smoking of cannabis are extremely rare. For patients with drug-induced psychosis, reassurance is usually sufficient. However, diazepam (0.1–0.2 mg / kg body weight i.v.) may be used for sedation if necessary. Hypotension usually responds well to intravenous fluids.

All patients who have injected cannabis should be admitted and careful management of fluid and electrolyte balance is essential owing to the risks of acute renal failure and pulmonary oedema.

Further reading

Brandenburg D, Wernick R. Intravenous marijuana syndrome. West Med J 1986; 145: 94–96.

MacNab A, Anderson E, Susak K. Ingestion of cannabis: A cause of coma in children. Pediatr Emerg Care 1989; 5: 238–239.

Strang J, Witton J, Hall W. Improving the quality of the cannabis debate: defining the different domains. BMJ 2000; 320: 108–110.

CARBAMAZEPINE

Used for the treatment of complex and simple partial seizures, trigeminal neuralgia and some psychiatric conditions.

Absorption is slow and unpredictable and it can take up to 6–24 hours for peak levels to be reached in overdose. Massive overdosage has been associated with the development of pharmacobezoars and the maximum serum concentrations may then not be attained until as late as 72 hours after ingestion. The half-life is also prolonged after massive overdose and is typically 30 hours. Carbamazepine undergoes enterohepatic recirculation and is metabolised to an active (10,11-epoxide) metabolite.

Clinical features

Acute poisoning is characterised by neurological features. Nystagmus, ataxia, intention tremor, fits and dysarthria are common. Confusion or aggression and impaired consciousness may also occur. Rarely, dizziness, mydriasis, divergent squint, dystonia, myoclonus, ophthalmoplegia and fixed dilated pupils have been described. Cardiological features such as sinus tachycardia, sino-atrial block, hypotension or hypertension are also common. Pancreatitis may occur but is very rare.

The most severe cases are characterised by CNS depression and marked tachycardia or bradycardia. Coma may be delayed for hours and be cyclical, as when the coma lightens, the gut wakes up and more drug is absorbed. Respiratory depression or apnoea can occur and pulmonary oedema occurs rarely. Fits can occur, particularly after massive overdose and some patients have died from persistent seizures. Death can also occur owing to cardiac arrhythmias or aspiration pneumonitis. Previous cardiovascular disease or age do *not* appear to be important prognostic factors.

> Warning! Severe cases are characterised by coma and severe tachycardia or bradycardia.

Essential investigations

Plasma concentrations of carbamazepine and the 10,11-epoxide, which is also toxic, can be measured by HPLC but do not correlate that well with toxicity, and are of limited use unless either sophisticated elimination methods are being used or identity of the drug taken is in doubt. Toxicity has been seen when serum concentrations exceed 20 mg/L (85 μmol/L), and when they exceed 40 mg/L (170 μmol/L) serious complications such as coma, fits, respiratory failure and conduction abnormalities tend to occur. Free serum carbamazepine concentrations may correlate better with clinical toxicity but are not widely available.

An ECG should be performed in all but the most trivial poisoning cases. First degree AV block, QRS prolongation and loss of P waves have been seen and carbamazepine overdose can make existing heart block worse.

> Warning! Carbamazepine levels are of little clinical value as they do not correlate well with severity of poisoning.
> Falling serum concentrations are not reassuring when the patient remains hypotensive and comatose.

Supportive care

Gastric lavage should be used if a patient presents within an hour of a massive overdose of carbamazepine (p. 9). Multiple-dose activated charcoal is indicated in symptomatic patients or after ingestion of >20 mg/kg and such elimination treatment can still be initiated within several hours of the overdose (p. 13).

Specific measures

Charcoal haemoperfusion increases carbamazepine clearance, but multiple doses of activated charcoal are almost as effective at achieving elimination of the drug. Charcoal haemoperfusion should be reserved for life-threatening toxicity (e.g. status epilepticus, cardiotoxicity), particularly if there is poor gut motility or renal impairment. Haemodialysis and peritoneal dialysis are not nearly as effective as charcoal haemoperfusion or multiple-dose charcoal.

Further reading
Jones AL, Proudfoot AT. Features and management of poisoning with modern drugs used to treat epilepsy. Q J Med 1998; 91: 325–332.

CHLOROQUINE

Chloroquine is used to prevent and treat malaria and in systemic lupus erythematosus and rheumatoid arthritis. Symptoms of overdose usually start within 1 hour of ingestion and include nausea, vomiting, agitation, drowsiness, hypokalaemia, headaches and visual disturbances. After large ingestions coma, convulsions, hypotension (due to a negative inotropic effect) and arrhythmias (widened QRS and QT intervals, ventricular tachycardia including torsades de pointes and ventricular fibrillation) occur.

Activated charcoal should be given (and gastric lavage considered) in all patients who present within 1 hour of ingestion of more than 15 mg/kg chloroquine. Avoid the use of antiarrhythmic agents if at all possible as this may precipitate further arrhythmias (p. 18). Overdrive pacing is the treatment of choice for ventricular dysrhythmias (p. 20). Inotropic support with adrenaline may be required (p. 17). Monitor plasma potassium – hypokalaemia may have a protective effect and should not be corrected in the early stages of poisoning. If hypokalaemia persists beyond 8 hours, replace potassium cautiously (rebound hyperkalaemia often occurs during the recovery phase). High dose diazepam (2 mg/kg body weight i.v. over 30 minutes) may have a protective effect in chloroquine poisoning, but respiratory support should be present before it is given.

CLOZAPINE

Clozapine is an atypical antipsychotic agent, used in the treatment of schizophrenia resistant to other agents. Clinical effects seen in overdose include drowsiness, confusion, agitation and extrapyramidal effects. Tachycardia, hypotension, arrhythmias, coma and respiratory depression can occur following large ingestions. Clozapine can cause agranulocytosis in therapy and although it has not been reported following overdose, all patients should have blood taken for a full blood count approximately 12 hours after ingestion. Patients should be observed with ECG monitoring for at least 12 hours after ingestion, or until asymptomatic. Extrapyramidal symptoms should be treated with procyclidine (adults: 5–10 mg i.v. or i.m. to a maximum of 20 mg/24 hours; children <2 years 0.5–2 mg, >2 years 2–5 mg, >10 years 5–10 mg i.m. or i.v., repeated after 20 minutes if necessary) or benztropine (adults: 1–2 mg i.m. or i.v. repeated as required; children: 20 μg/kg/dose i.m., i.v. or p.o.).

COCAINE/CRACK COCAINE

Cocaine (hydrochloride) is a white crystalline powder or colourless crystals. It is used clinically for vasoconstriction and anaesthesia of mucous membranes. As a street drug it may be sniffed into the nose (snorted) or injected intravenously, it is not smoked because it decomposes on heating. 'Crack' is cocaine, which has been separated from the hydrochloride base (free-base). It may be melted and smoked in a 'base' pipe or crushed, mixed with tobacco and smoked in a cigarette.

A typical 'line' of cocaine to be snorted contains 20–30 mg; crack is usually sold in 'rocks' containing 150 mg. The toxic dose is very variable and depends on individual tolerance, presence of other drugs and route of administration. However, ingestion of >1 g is potentially fatal.

Clinical features

After intranasal use the effects occur within minutes and may last 20–90 minutes. With intravenous use the peak 'high' occurs within 10 minutes. After oral intake the peak 'high' occurs within 45–90 minutes. Smoking 'crack' causes a peak 'high' within 10 minutes. In most cases the effects begin to resolve in about 20 minutes post-onset, except when taken intranasally. In fatal poisoning the onset and progression of symptoms is accelerated and death may occur in minutes. Survival beyond 3 hours indicates the patient is likely to survive.

Abuse of cocaine is followed by depression and dysphoria, which may lead to continual drug use. Binges may last 24–96 hours and end only when the patient becomes exhausted or runs out of cocaine. This depression is usually self-limiting and ends once the sleep pattern returns to normal.

Features of mild to moderate intoxication with cocaine include euphoria, agitation and aggression, slurred speech, ataxia, dilated pupils, restlessness, apprehension, bruxism (teeth grinding), nausea, vomiting, pallor, dizziness, headache, cold sweats, tremor, twitching, pyrexia, tachycardia, hallucinations (tactile, auditory, olfactory), ventricular ectopics, hypertension and increased respiration.

Features of severe intoxication include hyperreflexia, convulsions, incontinence and drowsiness. The respiration may be rapid and irregular with progressive hypoxia. Severe hypertension may cause haemorrhagic stroke. Coronary artery spasm may result in myocardial ischaemia or infarction even in patients with normal coronary arteries. Then hypotension, cyanosis and cardiac arrhythmias (VT/VF) occur. Hyperthermia associated with rhabdomyolysis, acute renal failure and disseminated intravascular coagulation (DIC) may occur. CNS depression, loss of reflexes, muscle paralysis, pulmonary oedema and circulatory and respiratory failure are also seen in severe poisoning.

Severe complications of cocaine use include:

- Stroke, including subarachnoid and intracerebral haemorrhage and cerebral infarcts.

- Cardiovascular complications; myocardial infarction, ventricular arrhythmias and cardiac arrest.
- Intestinal ischaemia.

Essential investigations

Patients with features of cocaine intoxication must have their blood pressure measured early and frequently and an ECG performed. Cocaine can be detected in the urine by simple drug of abuse screening tests (e.g. EMIT dipsticks) and by GC-MS. Metabolites of cocaine may be detected in the urine 2–3 days post-exposure. Cocaine is unstable in blood; samples need to be in fluoride oxalate tubes.

Supportive care

Give oral activated charcoal (adult 50 g, child 1 g/kg) within an hour of oral ingestion of any amount. All patients should be observed with ECG monitoring for a minimum of 2 hours. Monitor the blood pressure, heart rate, ECG and body temperature. Diazepam (0.1–0.2 mg/kg body weight) is useful for agitated or psychotic patients and it reduces central stimulation, which also reduces tachycardia, hypertension and pyrexia. Phenothiazines and haloperidol should be avoided for treatment of psychotic reactions because they can lower the threshold for convulsions.

Specific measures

For **cocaine-induced hypertension** the initial treatment of choice is diazepam (0.1–0.2 mg/kg body weight). If the diastolic BP remains greater than 140 mmHg and diazepam is ineffective in a patient who is otherwise reasonably well, nifedipine (5 mg sublingually for an adult) or oral alpha-blockers such as phenoxybenzamine or doxazosin may be given. If the diastolic BP is greater than 140 mmHg or the patient is showing any sign of hypertensive problems (e.g. encephalopathy, infarction, stroke, proteinuria) intravenous therapy is required. Agents that may be used include nitrates, alpha-blockers such as phentolamine and phenoxybenzamine, labetolol, or direct vasodilators such as sodium nitroprusside or hydralazine. These should be given to reduce the BP to under 200/110 mmHg as rapidly as possible. If the patient also has cardiac arrhythmias, intravenous verapamil (5–10 mg for an adult i.v.) may be the most appropriate drug.

The use of propranolol for treatment of cocaine-induced hypertension is controversial since it may itself cause hypertension due to unopposed alpha-stimulation. If this occurs, sodium nitroprusside (0.5 µg/kg/min by slow i.v. infusion in 5% glucose only) may be used to reverse propranolol-induced hypertensive crisis.

Cocaine-induced angina is a very complex management issue. Patients with chest pain after cocaine ingestion should be admitted to a Coronary Care Unit for ECG monitoring and further management. Intravenous or buccal nitrates are the treatment of choice. Calcium antagonists such as verapamil may also be used. Beta-blockers, particularly those with beta-2 effects (see p. 36), should be used with caution because of the risk of hypertension due to unopposed alpha-stimulation.

> Warning! In patients with a cocaine-induced myocardial infarction, use of thrombolytics is usually not necessary and should be considered carefully because the usual mechanism of cocaine-induced MI is spasm rather than thrombosis, and thrombolysis further increases the risk of intracranial haemorrhage. Expert cardiology and toxicology advice should be sought.

If the rectal temperature rises above 39°C, one litre of cold i.v. fluids should be given rapidly. Further fluid should be given according to clinical monitoring or CVP measurements. If a fluid challenge is ineffective in reducing the temperature then dantrolene is recommended (1 mg/kg i.v. over 10–15 minutes, if no response repeat the dose every 15 minutes to a maximum of 10 mg/kg in 24 hours). If there is still no response and especially in the presence of persistent convulsions, paralyse and ventilate.

Further reading

Goldfrank L, Hoffman R. The cardiovascular effects of cocaine. Ann Emerg Med 1991; 20: 165–175.

Hollander J. Cocaine associated myocardial infarction. JR Soc Med 1996; 89: 443–447.

LoVecchio F, Nelson L. Intraventricular bleeding after the use of thrombolytics in a cocaine user. Am J Emerg Med 1996; 14: 663–664.

CODEINE: see OPIOIDS

COLCHICINE

Colchicine is used in the treatment of gout and familial Mediterranean fever. Colchicine overdose can be associated with severe clinical effects and has a high mortality. There is often a delay of 6 hours before effects such as nausea, vomiting, abdominal pain and bloody diarrhoea occur. Gastrointestinal bleeding can be severe and result in hypotension and cardiovascular collapse. After 24 hours, confusion, drowsiness, coma, convulsions, acute renal failure, bone marrow hypoplasia, metabolic acidosis, arrhythmias and pulmonary oedema can occur. In severe cases multiple organ failure with bone marrow aplasia, acute renal failure, sepsis, ARDS, DIC and cerebral oedema can occur. Late complications include bone marrow suppression, alopecia, myopathy and peripheral neuropathy, all of which may persist for several weeks.

Multiple-dose activated charcoal (p. 13) should be given to adults who have ingested more than 0.1 mg/kg body weight and children who have ingested any amount. All patients should be observed for at least 6 hours post-ingestion – if they are asymptomatic at this stage they can be discharged with advice to return if gastrointestinal symptoms develop. Symptomatic patients should have blood taken for FBC, clotting, U&Es, liver function tests and creatine kinase, and should be placed on a cardiac monitor.

Further management depends on the subsequent clinical course. Patients who develop bone marrow suppression should be managed with input from a haematologist. Patients who develop significant GI symptoms should be followed up for 10–14 days with FBC, clotting, U&Es and liver function tests.

Haemodialysis and haemoperfusion are not of benefit.

DIGOXIN

Digoxin is a cardiac glycoside used in the treatment of atrial fibrillation and heart failure. Digitoxin is a related drug that is rarely used in the UK, it causes similar effects in overdose, the major difference being that it has a longer half-life (5–8 days). Cardiac glycosides are also found in plants, e.g. foxglove, oleander, lily of the valley and rhododendron.

Clinical features
Absorption of digoxin is slow and peak effects may be delayed up to 6–12 hours. The half-life of digoxin is 30–50 hours. Ingestion of $>50\,\mu g/kg$ body weight in a child or >2–3 mg in an adult is associated with toxicity. Patients who are already taking digoxin regularly and those with pre-existing cardiac disease are more susceptible to digoxin and smaller amounts can be toxic. Digoxin toxicity also occurs because of chronic accumulation in patients who are taking digoxin if the patient is on too high a dose, dehydrated, renally impaired, hypokalaemic or hypomagnesaemic (commonly because of diuretics). Digoxin toxicity may also be due to drug interactions with amiodarone, propafenone, calcium channel blockers or quinine (these all increase digoxin levels).

Clinical features
Nausea, vomiting and diarrhoea are common early features of digoxin poisoning. Other features include headache, confusion and more rarely visual effects and confusion. Hyperkalaemia is common in acute digoxin overdose and can be severe; it may also be seen in severe chronic poisoning. Digoxin poisoning can cause almost any type of heart block, bradyarrhythmia and tachyarrhythmia. The combination of tachyarrhythmias with heart block is particularly common. Severe poisoning is also associated with hypotension due to negative inotropic activity.

Essential investigations
U&E (hyperkalaemia can be severe, e.g. $>7\,mmol/L$). It is also important to document whether the patient has renal impairment. If possible a magnesium level is also helpful to exclude hypomagnesaemia, as it often occurs when hypokalaemia is present. A digoxin level is useful but not an absolute guide to toxicity, and clinical features are the best guide to the need for specific intervention.

Warning! All patients should have a 12-lead ECG.

Supportive care

All symptomatic patients should be on a cardiac monitor. Hyperkalaemia (potassium >5.5 mmol/L) should be treated with an insulin-dextrose infusion (50 ml 50% dextrose with 12 units of actrapid i.v. for an adult). Calcium gluconate/chloride should *NOT* be used to treat hyperkalaemia because it may worsen ventricular arrhythmias. Resistant or severe hyperkalaemia is an indication for digoxin-specific antibodies (see below).

Hypokalaemia or hypomagnesaemia should be treated with i.v. infusions. Sometimes inotropic support will be required and adrenaline or noradrenaline should be used (p. 17).

Specific measures

Activated charcoal (50 g in adults, 1 g/kg in children) should be given to all patients who present within an hour of the overdose. Use of further doses of activated charcoal (50 g 4-hourly) is controversial. Whilst it appears to increase digoxin elimination there is no clinical evidence that it alters patient outcome. However, we would advocate that multiple-dose activated charcoal be given to all patients with moderate-severe digoxin poisoning, on the grounds that it may interrupt the enterohepatic circulation of the drug and also bind residual digoxin within it.

Bradycardia with or without heart block *and* associated with haemodynamic compromise should be treated with atropine (adults: 0.6 mg i.v. repeated up to a maximum of 3 g; children 10–30 μg/kg). If the patient does not respond to atropine, digoxin-specific antibodies should be given. Temporary pacing or antiarrhythmic drugs should only be used if digoxin-specific antibodies are not immediately available because there is a risk of precipitating ventricular arrhythmias. The agents that can be considered for ventricular arrhythmias if digoxin-specific antibodies are not available are amiodarone (5 mg/kg body weight given centrally over 30 minutes) and phenytoin (15 mg/kg body weight i.v. at 50 mg/minute). DC cardioversion should be avoided if possible because of the risk of precipitating asystole or VF. When absolutely necessary it should be attempted using lower energy settings (25–50 J) and synchronised.

Fab fragments of digoxin-specific antibodies are indicated in **severe poisoning**, i.e. in the following circumstances:

- Severe hyperkalaemia (>6.0 mmol/L) resistant to treatment with insulin-dextrose infusion.
- Bradycardia or heart block associated with hypotension resistant to treatment with atropine.
- Tachyarrhythmias associated with hypotension (particularly ventricular arrhythmias).

They should be considered at less severe stages of poisoning in the elderly and those with previous cardiovascular disease. Fab fragments are usually well tolerated (very rarely a serum sickness reaction may be seen) and improvement is seen within 10–30 minutes of their use. The dose given can be calculated from either the dose of digoxin ingested or the serum digoxin concentration.

Number of 40 mg vials of Fab = Serum digoxin concentration (ng/ml) × body weight × 0.0084

OR

Number of 40 mg vials of Fab = Ingested dose (mg) × 1.2

If neither of these is known, we would advise giving 10–20 vials of 40 mg Fab and repeating this dose if necessary after 2–4 hours.

The Fab fragment should be given as an infusion over 30 minutes, but can be given as a bolus for immediately life-threatening arrhythmias. U&Es should be checked 2–4 hours after starting Fab fragments because of the risk of hypokalaemia.

> Warning! Patients with digoxin poisoning can deteriorate rapidly – make sure that Fab fragments are available, don't wait for VT/heart block to develop.

Further reading

Lip GYH, Metcalfe MJ, Dunn FG. Diagnosis and treatment of digoxin toxicity. Postgrad Med J 1993; 69: 337–339.

Taboulet P, Baud FJ, Bismuth C. Clinical features and management of digitalis poisoning – rationale for immunotherapy. Clin Toxicol 1993; 31(2): 247–260.

DIHYDROCODEINE: see OPIOIDS

ECSTASY/AMPHETAMINES

MDMA (3,4-methylenedioxymethamphetamine) is an amphetamine derivative. It is classified as a Class A drug under the Misuse of Drugs Act 1971. Ecstasy produces stimulation of the sympathetic nervous system both centrally and peripherally and also prevents re-uptake of catecholamines, dopamine and serotonin. Slang terms (p. 141) include E, Adam, White Dove, Denis the Menace, White burger, Red and Black.

> Warning! Many substances are now added to ecstasy tablets such as caffeine and ketamine. There is current vogue for using sildafenil (Viagra) together with ectasy for enhanced effects, so-called 'sexstasy'.

Clinical features

The half-life of MDMA is 7.6 hours. Effects occur within 1 hour and last 4–6 hours following doses of 75–150 mg and up to 48 hours after 100–300 mg. However, tolerance is common, and most users need to take considerably higher doses after several weeks of use.

Cardiac arrhythmias are common and deaths, which occur soon after ingestion, are usually due to cardiac arrhythmias. Arrhythmias are usually supraventricular, though ventricular ones occur also. Agitation or drowsiness are common. Whilst the vast majority of ecstasy patients are profoundly dehydrated a small proportion develop hyponatraemia, usually after drinking excessive amounts of water in the absence of sufficient exertion to sweat off the fluid. Anti-diuretic hormone secretion may be responsible.

Other features include nausea, hypertonia, hyperreflexia, muscle pain, trismus (jaw-clenching), dilated pupils, blurred vision, sweating, dry mouth, agitation, visual hallucinations, anxiety, hypertension, tachycardia. Severe intoxication is characterised by coma, convulsions, hypertension or hypotension and cardiac dysrhythmias (supraventricular more commonly than ventricular). Severe hypertension may cause haemorrhagic stroke. Fulminant hepatic failure has been reported after ecstasy ingestion.

A hyperthermic (serotonin-like) syndrome (p. 25) may develop with rigidity, hyperreflexia and hyperpyrexia (over 39°C) leading to hypotension, rhabdomyolysis, metabolic acidosis, acute renal failure, disseminated intravascular coagulation (DIC), hepatocellular necrosis, adult respiratory distress syndrome and cardiovascular collapse.

Essential investigations

U&Es, creatine kinase, full blood count, liver function tests, blood glucose. An ECG is required. MDMA levels in blood do not correlate with clinical signs and are not of value in management.

Supportive care

Activated charcoal (adult: 50 g, child: 1 g/kg) can be considered up to 1 hour post-ingestion. Observe all cases with ECG monitoring for at least 6 hours post-exposure. Monitor BP, heart rate, ECG and body temperature.

Diazepam (0.1–0.2 mg/kg body weight) is useful for agitated or psychotic patients and it reduces central stimulation, which also reduces tachycardia, hypertension and pyrexia. Haloperidol should be avoided as it can lower the threshold for convulsions, although it may be used if diazepam is ineffective to help control an agitated patient.

Specific measures

Supraventricular tachycardia should be treated with verapamil or beta-1 selective blockers such as esmolol or metoprolol (p. 18). Propranolol should not be used because it can cause hypertension due to unopposed alpha-stimulation.

Hypertension: The initial treatment of choice is diazepam (0.1–0.2 mg/kg body weight). If the diastolic BP remains greater than 140 mmHg and diazepam is ineffective in a patient who is otherwise reasonably well, nifedipine (5 mg sublingually for an adult) or oral alpha-blockers such as phenoxybenzamine or doxazosin may be given. If the diastolic BP is greater than 140 mmHg or the patient is showing any sign of hypertensive problems (e.g. encephalopathy, infarction, stroke, proteinuria) intravenous therapy is required. Agents that may be used include nitrates, alpha-blockers such as phentolamine and phenoxybenzamine, and labetolol. Alternatively, direct vasodilators such as sodium nitroprusside or hydralazine should be given to reduce the BP to less than 200/110 mmHg as rapidly as possible.

Hyperthermia: If the rectal temperature exceeds 39°C, at least one litre of cold intravenous fluid should be given rapidly, further fluid should be given according to clinical parameters or CVP measurements. If a fluid challenge is ineffective in reducing the temperature then dantrolene should be used (1 mg/kg i.v. over 10–15 minutes – if there is no response repeat this dose every 15 minutes to a maximum of 10 mg/kg in 24 hours). If this is ineffective the patient should be paralysed and ventilated. In the future specific serotonergic agents may be used in patients with serotonin syndrome, e.g. cyproheptadine/ketanserin to reduce temperature and rigidity by central mechanisms (p. 25).

Further reading

Maxwell DL, Polkey MI, Henry JA. Hyponatraemia and catatonic stupor after taking ecstasy. BMJ 1993; 307: 1399.

Denborough MA, Hopkinson KC. Dantrolene and 'ecstasy'. Med J Austr 1997; 166: 165–166.

Henry JA, Jeffreys KJ, Dawling S. Toxicity and deaths from 3,4-methylenedioxymethamphetamine ('ecstasy'). Lancet 1992; 340: 384–387.

Jones AL, Simpson K. Mechanisms and management of hepatotoxicity in ecstasy (MDMA) and amphetamine intoxications. Alimen Pharmacol 1999; 12: 129–133.

GAMMAHYDROXYBUTYRIC ACID (GHB)

GHB is marketed illegally for bodybuilding, weight loss, as a psychedelic drug and as a replacement for L-tryptophan. GHB is sold as the sodium salt, either in powder or granular form, often presented in a capsule. It is commonly dissolved in water to produce a clear colourless liquid. The taste is similar to that of seaweed.

GHB is a controlled drug under the Medicines Act, and manufacture and distribution is an offence. However, it is not controlled under the Misuse of Drugs Act and possession is not illegal. Slang terms include Liquid X, Cherry Meth, Easy Lay, Scoop and GBH (see p. 141).

As the drug is taken in liquid form it is difficult to estimate the correct dose, so many abusers simply 'guzzle' it until they reach an adequate high. This is often achieved shortly before becoming unconscious. The effects of

GHB have been likened to a combination of ecstasy and LSD, but owing to the drowsiness that may occur, it is sometimes mixed with amphetamines to prolong the 'high' for several hours.

Clinical features

The severity and duration of effects seem to be dependent on dose. 10–30 mg/kg: mild effects such as nausea, diarrhoea, confusion, vertigo, tremor, extrapyramidal signs, agitation and euphoria. 50 mg/kg: drowsiness, coma, bradycardia, hypotension, Cheyne-Stokes respiration. >50 mg/kg: decreased cardiac output and increasingly severe respiratory depression, fits and coma. The effects are potentiated by other CNS depressants (e.g. alcohol, benzodiazepines, opioids and neuroleptic drugs).

The response to low oral doses of GHB is unpredictable, with variation in CNS depression in the same patient and between patients. No fatalities due to GHB alone have been reported, although many cases that present to hospital require emergency supportive care. Bizarrely, patients often recover quickly within 1–2 hours with scenarios such as self-extubation and rapid reversal of coma seen in intensive care. Coma usually resolves spontaneously within 2–4 hours, but rarely may persist for as long as 96 hours. Most users feel 'high' for 24–48 hours and then suffer a hung-over state for a further 48–72 hours. Dizziness may last for up to 2 weeks.

Essential investigations

U&Es and glucose should be measured in all but the most trivial of cases. Metabolic acidosis, hypernatraemia, hypokalaemia and hyperglycaemia can occur. GHB concentrations in plasma are not recommended routinely.

Supportive care

Activated charcoal treatment is recommended for more than 20 mg/kg body weight in adults or any amount in a child up to 1 hour after ingestion. All patients should be observed for a minimum of 2 hours, with monitoring of blood pressure, heart rate, and respiratory rate and oxygenation. Patients symptomatic after this time should be admitted and observed until symptoms resolve. They will require supportive care only.

Naloxone has been shown to reverse some of the effects of GHB in animals but the efficacy in humans has not been studied. Diazepam is the drug of choice for convulsions (0.1–0.2 mg/kg body weight). Bradycardia may be controlled with i.v. atropine (0.6–1.2 mg for an adult, 0.02 mg/kg for a child).

Further reading

Dyer JE. Gamma-hydroxybutyrate: A health food product producing coma and seizure-like activity. Am J Emerg Med 1991; 9: 321–324.

Bismuth C, Dally S, Borron SW. Chemical submission: GHB, benzodiazepines and other knockout drops. Clin Toxicol 1997; 35: 595–598.

HALOPERIDOL AND OTHER BUTYROPHENONES

Haloperidol is a butyrophenone antipsychotic agent (others include droperidol and benperidol, which cause similar effects when taken in overdose). In overdose haloperidol causes drowsiness, and extrapyramidal effects are also common including tremor, rigidity and acute dystonic reactions. Rarely hypotension, QT prolongation, arrhythmias and convulsions may develop.

Activated charcoal should be given, and gastric lavage considered, for patients who present within 1 hour of ingestion of more than 200 mg (10 mg in children). Extrapyramidal symptoms should be treated with procyclidine (adults: 5–10 mg i.v. or i.m. to a maximum of 20 mg/24 hours; children <2 years: 0.5–2 mg, >2 years: 2–5 mg, >10 years: 5–10 mg i.m. or i.v., repeated after 20 minutes if necessary) or benztropine (adults: 1–2 mg i.m. or i.v. repeated as required; children: 20 µg/kg/dose i.m., i.v. or p.o.).

All patients should be observed for 6 hours after ingestion; patients who remain symptomatic at this stage should be observed for 24 hours post-ingestion with ECG monitoring. Ventricular arrhythmias, if they occur, should be treated with cardioversion, phenytoin or lignocaine (p. 19). In severe cases, or if torsade de pointes develops, arrhythmias may be unresponsive to both drug therapy and cardioversion, and transvenous pacing is necessary (p. 20).

Warning! Class Ia antiarrhythmics are contraindicated.

HEROIN: see OPIOIDS

INSULIN: see ANTIDIABETIC AGENTS

IRON

Iron and iron salts are used for the treatment or prophylaxis of iron deficiency anaemia. Oral iron preparations may be tablets or capsules in immediate-release or modified-release form, or liquids. Parenteral preparations are also available. Iron is also available in combination with folic acid and vitamins and so if a patient takes an overdose of an over-the-counter vitamin preparation it is important to check the iron content. There are many different iron preparations, which contain different amounts of elemental iron (Table 2.2).

Clinical features
The early features of iron poisoning are due to the corrosive effects of iron, while later effects are largely due to the disruption of cellular processes. Iron tablets may adhere to the stomach or duodenum causing irritation and in severe cases haemorrhagic necrosis and perforation. The consequent fluid and blood loss may be substantial and result in severe hypovolaemia. This in turn results in tissue hypoxia, lactic acidosis and circulatory collapse.

Absorbed iron is rapidly cleared from the extracellular space by uptake into parenchymal cells, particularly in the liver. It causes mitochondrial

TABLE 2.2 Elemental iron content of iron preparations

Iron preparation	Usual dosage	Amount of **elemental** iron
Ferrous fumarate	200 mg	65 mg
Ferrous gluconate	300 mg	35 mg
Ferrous succinate	100 mg	35 mg
Ferrous sulphate	200 mg	60 mg
Ferrous sulphate (dried)	300 mg	60–65 mg

Toxic doses of **elemental** iron are:
< 30 mg/kg: mild toxicity
> 30 mg/kg: moderate toxicity
> 60 mg/kg: severe toxicity
> 150 mg/kg: lethal

damage and cellular dysfunction resulting in metabolic acidosis and necrosis. Eventually widespread organ damage becomes apparent, hepatic failure with hypoglycaemia and coagulopathy may develop and this is often fatal.

The **clinical course** of iron poisoning may be divided into four phases; the time scale is variable.

Phase 1: From 30 minutes to several hours after ingestion, effects are due to the corrosive effects of iron. Vomiting/haematemesis, diarrhoea, melaena and abdominal pain occur. The vomit and stools may smell metallic. In severe cases gastrointestinal haemorrhage can result in shock, metabolic acidosis and renal failure.

Phase 2: 6–24 hours after ingestion the clinical effects usually abate and the patient either recovers or moves on to the next phase.

Warning! In severe cases this phase may not be apparent or a latent phase occurs and is deceptively reassuring.

Phase 3: 12–48 hours after ingestion severe lethargy, coma, convulsions, gastrointestinal haemorrhage, shock, cardiovascular collapse, metabolic acidosis, hepatic failure with hypoglycaemia, coagulopathy, pulmonary oedema and renal failure may occur.

Phase 4: At 2–5 weeks, scarring from the initial corrosive damage can result in small bowel strictures and pyloric stenosis.

Essential investigations
Blood should be taken at 4 hours post-ingestion for determination of the **serum iron level**. If desferrioxamine is to be given before 4 hours because of severe poisoning then blood should be taken for determination of the serum iron level just prior to its administration. Once desferrioxamine has been given, colorimetric assay methods may underestimate the amount of free

serum iron and atomic absorption spectrophotometry is a more accurate analytical method. A blood level taken more than 4 hours after ingestion may underestimate the amount of free iron because of distribution into tissues. However, for sustained-release preparations an initial serum level should be taken at 4 hours and again at 6–8 hours post-ingestion. The serum iron concentration should be determined on arrival for late presenting patients. In such patients a low concentration cannot be interpreted, a high concentration would indicate toxicity.

> **Warning!** It is essential to interpret the iron level in the context of the patient's clinical condition and an accurate patient history. The iron concentration cannot be interpreted in isolation.
> Measurement of the total iron binding capacity is of no value and should not be undertaken.

Further treatment should be determined by the patient's clinical condition and the serum iron concentration.

The following serum iron levels (Table 2.3) give a *rough guide* to the expected severity:

TABLE 2.3   Serum iron levels and toxicity

<55 µmol/L (<300 µg/100 ml)	Mild toxicity
55–90 µmol/L (300–500 µg/100 ml)	Moderate toxicity
>90 µmol/L (500 µg/100 ml)	Severe toxicity
>180 µmol/L (1000 µg/100 ml)	Potentially lethal

All patients should also have blood taken for FBC (leucocytosis is common), U&Es, glucose (hyperglycaemia is common), liver function tests and clotting. Arterial blood gases should be checked in symptomatic or severely poisoned patients. If serum iron concentrations are not available, the presence of nausea, vomiting, leucocytosis ($>15 \times 10^9$/L) and hyperglycaemia (>8.3 mmol/L) suggests significant ingestion.

Supportive care
After ingestion of <30 mg/kg of elemental iron patients are unlikely to require active treatment, but may develop vomiting. If this is severe, rehydration may be necessary.

After ingestion of >30 mg/kg of elemental iron an **abdominal X-ray** should be performed to determine the need for gut decontamination. Undissolved iron tablets are radiopaque: if any are visible on X-ray then gastric lavage (if tablets are seen in the stomach), using as wide-bore a tube as possible, or whole bowel irrigation (if tablets are seen in the small bowel) with polyethylene glycol, should be undertaken (p. 12). Iron tablets that have dissolved are not radiopaque.

> Warning! Iron tablets are not bound to activated charcoal.
> The absence of radiopaque material on X-ray does not eliminate the possibility of ingestion.

Rehydrate with intravenous fluids and replace blood if necessary, but be careful to avoid fluid overload because there is a risk of pulmonary oedema.

Specific measures

Parenteral desferrioxamine chelates free iron, removing it from cellular binding sites. The decision to use it should be based on the patient's clinical condition and on laboratory analyses.

● Patients with a serum iron level of 55–90 μmol/L (300–500 μg/100 ml) should be observed for 24–48 hours post-ingestion. They do not require chelation therapy unless they develop symptoms or have haematemesis or melaena.
● i.v. desferrioxamine should be given *urgently* to patients with hypotension, shock, severe lethargy, coma or convulsions, or a serum iron level of >90 μmol/L (>500 μg/100 ml).

Dosage of desferrioxamine is 15 mg/kg/hour (this may be reduced after 2–4 hours), up to a maximum of 80 mg/kg in 24 hours. Doses of >80 mg/kg have been used but should first be discussed with a clinical toxicologist. Desferrioxamine can be given i.m. but this route is not recommended for the treatment of iron poisoning because a large volume needs to be injected and this is painful. Also absorption by this route may be irregular, particularly if the patient is hypotensive.

> Warning! If intravenous desferrioxamine is given at a faster rate than 15 mg/kg/hour it may cause hypotension.
> If more than 80 mg/kg is given i.v. over 24 hours, pulmonary complications such as ARDS may ensue.

Desferrioxamine should be given until all the following have happened: urine has returned to a normal colour, symptoms have abated, and all radio-opacities have disappeared. Haemodialysis may be needed to remove the iron-desferrioxamine complex in patients with renal failure.

Further reading

Klein-Schwartz W, Oderda GM, Gorman RL, Favin F, Rose SR. Assessment of management guidelines. Acute iron ingestion. Clin Pediatr 1990; 29(6): 316–321.

Proudfoot AT, Simpson D, Dyson EH. Management of acute iron poisoning. Med Toxicol 1986; 1(2): 83–100.

Tenenbein M. Benefits of parenteral desferrioxamine for acute iron poisoning. Clin Toxicol 1996; 34(5): 485–489.

ISONIAZID

Isoniazid is an antituberculous drug which is often used in combination with other drugs. It is rapidly absorbed and peak levels occur within 1–2 hours. The half-life is 1–2 hours in fast acetylators and 2–5 hours in slow acetylators; the half-life is also increased in patients with hepatic or renal dysfunction. Fast acetylators have an average plasma concentration 30–50% of that in slow acetylators.

Clinical features

Doses of $>15–20$ mg/kg result in mild toxicity, >80 mg/kg in severe toxicity and >150 mg/kg is potentially fatal if not managed appropriately.

Mild features include nausea and vomiting, tachycardia, dizziness, hallucinations, increased visual sensitivity (coloured lights and spots), hyperreflexia and pyrexia.

Severe poisoning is characterised by coma, respiratory depression, hypotension and convulsions which may progress to status epilepticus, together with the development of a severe high anion gap metabolic acidosis. Rhabomyolysis may develop in patients with protracted convulsions and may cause acute renal failure. Permanent neurological damage may result from isoniazid toxicity.

> **Warning!** Acute isoniazid poisoning is characterised by refractory convulsions, severe metabolic acidosis and coma.

Supportive care

Activated charcoal should be given if >15 mg/kg has been ingested within the last 1 hour. Gastric lavage followed by activated charcoal should be considered for ingestions of >80 mg/kg within the last 1 hour. The patient should be observed for at least 6 hours post-ingestion. Ventilation may be required in severe cases.

Specific measures

Pyridoxine is a specific antidote for isoniazid overdose. Convulsions should be controlled with diazepam (0.1–0.2 mg/kg body weight) *and* pyridoxine, which act synergistically. Pyridoxine should be given at a dose of 1 g pyridoxine i.v. for every gram of isoniazid ingested to a maximum of 5 g in adults (where the dose of isoniazid is unknown give 5 g of pyridoxine) and in children at a dose of 70 mg/kg to a maximum of 5 g. Administration of pyridoxine should also be considered in an asymptomatic patient with a good history of ingestion of a toxic quantity (particularly if >80 mg/kg). The earlier pyridoxine is started, the fewer the complications. Thiopentone may be used for refractory convulsions.

Isoniazid has poor protein binding and a low volume of distribution and is therefore a good candidate for removal by haemodialysis, but because of the short half-life and effective control of convulsions with pyridoxine/ diazepam this is rarely required. It should be considered in cases not responding to supportive care or in patients with renal insufficiency.

KETAMINE

Ketamine is a parenteral general anaesthetic agent with analgesic properties, used in both human and veterinary medicine. When used as an anaesthetic it produces 'dissociative' anaesthesia. Illicit preparations are available as capsules, crystals and powders for sniffing or smoking. Slang terms include Special K, Kit-Kat, Super K and Vitamin K.

Clinical features
Onset of effects is rapid, within minutes, and the psychological effects usually last 30–60 minutes.

Mild effects after ingestion include euphoria, agitation and aggression, vomiting, slurred speech, blurred vision, numbness, dizziness and ataxia. Moderate effects include hypertension and tachycardia; patients are often very aggressive. The feeling of dissociation can be very dramatic – there are many reports of 'out of body' experiences. Other psychological effects include synaesthesia ('seeing' sounds and 'hearing' colours), depersonalisation, stereotypies (persistent repetition of actions or words) and confusion. As the patient comes round, an 'emergence reaction' is often experienced, characterised by floating sensations, vivid dreams (pleasant or unpleasant), often hypersensitivity to light, hallucinations and delirium.

Severe effects include convulsions, polyneuropathy, raised intracranial pressure, pulmonary oedema, respiratory depression, cardiac and respiratory arrest.

Essential investigations
Oxygen saturation should be monitored if breathing is compromised.

Supportive care
All patients should be observed for a minimum of 4 hours. Activated charcoal may be given within 1 hour of ingestion if an oral preparation has been taken. The patient should be placed in a quiet, calm environment. Monitor BP, pulse and respiration. Diazepam (0.1–0.2 mg/kg body weight) may be given for agitation and panic attacks and also as treatment for convulsions, but should be used with caution owing to its respiratory depressant effect.

Specific measures
The 'emergence reaction' responds to diazepam (0.1–0.2 mg/kg body weight). Minimising external stimuli is also important in these patients.

Further reading
Jansen KLR. Non-medical use of ketamine. BMJ 1993; 306: 601–602.

LAMOTRIGINE

Used for treatment of partial seizures and secondary generalised tonic–clonic seizures unresponsive to treatment with other anticonvulsants.

Clinical features
Large overdoses can be associated with sedation, ataxia, diplopia, nausea and vomiting. Hypertonia, nystagmus and widening of QRS on ECG have also been seen.

Essential investigations
There is no value in measuring the drug concentration in blood. If serious toxicity is possible, an ECG should be done.

Supportive care
Activated charcoal should be given (and gastric lavage considered) in all adults who present within an hour of ingestion of more than 10 tablets.

Specific measures
None.

Further reading
Jones AL, Proudfoot AT. Features and management of poisoning with modern drugs used to treat epilepsy. Q J Med 1998; 91: 325–332.

LITHIUM

Lithium is used in the treatment and prophylaxis of mania, manic-depressive illness and recurrent depression. It is also used in the treatment of aggressive or self-mutilating behaviour. It is available as sustained-release tablets (the most commonly prescribed), non-sustained-release tablets and liquid.

Clinical features
A single acute overdose usually carries low risk and patients tend to show mild symptoms independent of serum lithium concentrations. More severe symptoms may occur after a delay if lithium elimination is impaired. However, if a patient on chronic lithium therapy has taken an acute overdose, this can lead to serious toxicity. Lithium toxicity can also occur as a result of chronic accumulation if the patient has been on too high a dose or is dehydrated, or if a drug interaction takes place (thiazide diuretics, NSAIDs, ACE inhibitors, tetracycline all increase lithium levels). In patients with raised lithium levels, the risk of toxicity is greater in those with hypertension, diabetes, congestive heart failure, chronic renal failure, schizophrenia and Addison's disease.

After ingestion of liquid lithium, peak levels occur after 30 minutes. With sustained-release tablets absorption is variable and peak levels occur after 4–5 hours. Half-life ranges from 8–45 hours (mean 24 hours); this may be prolonged in overdose. The onset of symptoms may be delayed for up to 24 hours especially in lithium-naive patients.

- Mild features: Nausea, diarrhoea, blurred vision, polyuria, light-headedness, fine tremor, muscular weakness and drowsiness.
- Moderate features: Increasing confusion, blackouts, fasciculation and hyperreflexia. Myoclonic twitches and jerks, choreoathetoid movements, urinary or faecal incontinence, increasing restlessness followed by stupor. Hypernatraemia.
- Severe features: Coma, convulsions, cardiac arrhythmias including sino-atrial block, sinus and junctional bradycardia and heart block, hypotension or rarely hypertension, and renal failure. Patients recovering from lithium intoxication may have neurological sequelae (cerebellar signs).

Supportive care and specific measures
See flowchart 2.1 for full details.

   Gut decontamination: Activated charcoal does not bind lithium and so should only be used if other drugs have been co-ingested. The method used for gut decontamination depends on the type of preparation that has been taken. For liquid lithium preparations, nasogastric aspiration should be used if the patient presents within 1 hour of ingestion. If the patient has taken non-sustained-release lithium tablets, gastric lavage should be considered if the patient presents within 1 hour of ingestion. However, sustained-release lithium tablets are too large to pass up a lavage tube and the method of choice for overdose with these tablets is whole bowel irrigation (see p. 12 for method).

   Lithium levels: These should be taken at presentation in cases of chronic accumulation and at 6 hours post-ingestion for acute and acute-on-chronic overdose. The lithium level is not an absolute predictor of toxicity, particularly in chronic accumulation and acute-on-chronic overdose. Lithium levels should be repeated 6–12-hourly in symptomatic patients until clinical improvement occurs. They should also be repeated if a sustained release preparation has been taken.

   Meticulous supportive care and monitoring is important in patients with lithium poisoning. All symptomatic patients should be on a cardiac monitor. Patients should be rehydrated, and fluid balance and U&Es monitored. Diazepam (0.1–0.2 mg/kg body weight) is the treatment of choice for convulsions. Patients should be observed for a minimum of 24 hours.

   Haemodialysis: Lithium is effectively removed by haemodialysis. Haemodialysis is indicated in all patients with severe lithium poisoning, i.e. coma, convulsions, respiratory failure or acute renal failure. Lithium levels can also be used to guide the need for haemodialysis (see flowchart 2.1) although as mentioned above they are not an absolute guide to toxicity. Lower thresholds for haemodialysis should be used in patients with renal impairment. Haemodialysis should be continued for 6–12 hours; generally

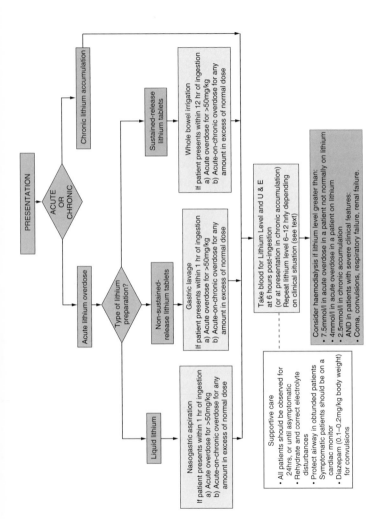

Fig. 2.1 Lithium overdose

each hour of dialysis will reduce the plasma lithium concentration by 1 mmol/L. Lithium levels often rebound after haemodialysis and so levels should be repeated at the end of dialysis and again 6–12 hours later.

Haemofiltration: The use of CVVHF/CAVHF has been reported in patients with lithium poisoning. However, the evidence for effective lithium removal by haemofiltration is limited and so haemodialysis is still the treatment of choice in patients with lithium poisoning.

> Warning! Don't take blood for a lithium level in a lithium-heparin tube – this will give falsely high levels.

Further reading

Jaeger A, Sauder P, Kopferschmitt J, Tritsch L, Flesch F. When should dialysis be performed in lithium poisoning? A kinetic study in 14 cases of lithium poisoning. Clin Toxicol 1993; 31: 429–447.

Leblanc M, Raymond M, Bonnardeaux A, Isenring P, Pichette V, Geadah D, Ouimet D, Ethier J, Cardinal J. Lithium poisoning treated by high-performance continuous arterio-venous and veno-venous hemodiafiltration. Am J Kidney Diseases 1996; 27: 365–372.

LYSERGIC ACID DIETHYLAMIDE (LSD)

d-Lysergic acid diethylamide (LSD) is a synthetic hallucinogen which is currently classified as a Class A drug under the 1971 Misuse of Drugs Act. Common slang terms are acid, trips, dots, paper mushrooms or 'L'. LSD is usually ingested as small squares of impregnated absorbent paper, which are often printed with a distinctive design, or as 'microdots', i.e. very small LSD tablets. It may also be taken in capsule or tablet form. A 'normal street dose' is around 50–70 µg. Intravenous, nasal (snorting), and pulmonary (smoking) methods of abuse are rare.

Clinical features

Patients rarely appear in hospital with LSD intoxication. Those who do usually do so as a result of a 'bad-trip', panic reaction, hallucinations, aggression or after a suicide attempt. The individual may be found wandering in a confused, agitated state. Dilated pupils are common.

Peak plasma concentrations and peak effects are seen within 30–60 minutes of an oral dose of 2 µg/kg, and within 15–30 minutes following i.v. administration, and the serum half-life in man is approximately 3 hours. Tolerance occurs after 4–5 days.

LSD itself is of low acute toxicity; fatalities are a result of behavioural changes induced by LSD leading to accidents such as drowning. In rare cases snorting has resulted in coma, bleeding, and severe pyrexia, although all patients recovered fully. Features of mild intoxication include nausea, vomiting, dilated pupils, salivation, lacrimation, weakness, tremor, ataxia and hyperreflexia. With increased intoxication tachycardia, tachypnoea, and mild pyrexia can occur. Anxiety, paranoia, depersonalisation, variable behavioural changes, hyperacusis and auditory hallucinations are common. Whilst spatial and colour distortions are common, frank visual hallucinations are rare. Severe features are rarely seen as a result of non-oral abuse and include coma, convulsions, pyrexia, and GI bleeding, probably due to inhibition of platelet aggregation.

Flashbacks can occur within hours or months after acute or chronic abuse. These may be precipitated by physical or emotional stress.

Essential investigations
None.

Supportive care
Activated charcoal is unlikely to be necessary unless it is a child who presents within 1 hour of ingestion (give 1 g/kg). Patients showing psychotic reactions or CNS depression should be observed in hospital. Minimise external stimuli by placing the patient in a dimly lit, quiet room. Reassure by talking to the patient. Where sedation is required, diazepam (0.1–0.2 mg/kg i.v.) is the drug of choice. Haloperidol (5–10 mg orally) can be considered for psychotic reactions if diazepam is ineffective. Other phenothiazines should be used cautiously, chlorpromazine has been associated with cardiovascular collapse in LSD intoxication.

Specific measures
None required.

Further reading
Klock JC. Coma, hyperthermia and bleeding associated with massive LSD overdose: A report of eight cases. Clin Toxicol 1997; 8: 191–203.

MONOAMINE–OXIDASE INHIBITORS (MAOIs)

Monoamine-oxidase inhibitors (MAOIs) are used in the treatment of depression. There are three of the original MAOIs that are still available in the UK: phenelzine, tranylcypromine and isocarboxazid. Moclobemide is a newer, reversible monoamine-oxidase inhibitor that appears to be less hazardous than the other agents in overdose.

Clinical features
In overdose the clinical features may be delayed for 6–24 hours and may persist for several days. Anxiety, restlessness, confusion, flushing, sweating, headache, vomiting, tremor, myoclonus and hyperreflexia are common in mild intoxication. Less commonly there is hyperventilation, hypertension and tachycardia. In severe intoxication, severe hypertension (which can lead to intracranial haemorrhage), delirium, coma, hyperthermia, rigidity, opisthotonus and metabolic acidosis can occur. Complications include rhabdomyolysis, acute renal failure and disseminated intravascular coagulation (DIC).

Supportive care

Gastric lavage followed by 50 g activated charcoal if ingestion of more than five tablets in an adult has taken place within the last 1 hour. Cardiac monitoring should be instituted for 24 hours for all but the most trivial overdose. Diazepam can be given for sedation if necessary.

Specific measures

Hypertension: The initial treatment of choice is diazepam (0.1–0.2 mg/kg body weight). If the diastolic BP remains greater than 140 mmHg and diazepam is ineffective in a patient who is otherwise reasonably well, nifedipine (5 mg sublingually for an adult), or oral alpha-blockers such as phenoxybenzamine or doxazosin, may be given. If the diastolic BP is greater than 140 mmHg or the patient is showing any sign of hypertensive problems (e.g. encephalopathy, infarction, stroke, proteinuria) then intravenous therapy is required. Intravenous agents, e.g. nitrates, alpha-blockers such as phentolamine and phenoxybenzamine, labetolol, or direct vasodilators such as sodium nitroprusside or hydralazine should be given to reduce the BP to under 200/110 mmHg as rapidly as possible. Propranolol should not be used because it can cause worse hypertension due to unopposed alpha-stimulation.

Hyperthermia: If the rectal temperature exceeds 39°C, at least 1 litre of cold intravenous fluid should be given rapidly; further fluid should be given according to clinical parameters or CVP measurements. If a fluid challenge is ineffective in reducing the temperature then dantrolene should be used (1 mg/kg i.v. over 10–15 minutes; if there is no response repeat this dose every 15 minutes to a maximum of 10 mg/kg in 24 hours). If this is ineffective the patient should be paralysed and ventilated. Monitor U&Es, creatine kinase and check for DIC.

Serotonin syndrome (p. 25) may be caused by interaction between MAOIs and many drugs including SSRIs, dextromorphan and tricyclic antidepressants.

METFORMIN: see ANTIDIABETIC AGENTS

MORPHINE: see OPIOIDS

NON-STEROIDAL ANTI-INFLAMMATORY DRUGS (NSAIDs)

Mefenamic acid and ibuprofen are very commonly taken in overdose.

Clinical features

Overdose by most NSAIDs causes little more than mild gastrointestinal upset including mild abdominal pain. Vomiting and diarrhoea may occur owing to the cyclo-oxygenase inhibiting action of the drugs. 10–20% of patients taking a NSAID overdose (particularly of mefenamic acid) may have convulsions, which are usually self-limiting and seldom need treatment other than airway protection and oxygen. Acidosis may rarely occur with large ingestions. Drowsiness, lethargy, ataxia, nystagmus, blurred vision and tachycardia may rarely occur. Serious features include coma, prolonged fits, apnoea and bradycardia, but are very rare. Deaths have been reported after massive overdose of ibuprofen, but none so far with mefenamic acid. Rarely, renal failure ensues and therefore urea and electrolytes should be checked in large ingestions.

Essential laboratory investigations
Although NSAID drug concentrations in plasma can be measured in toxicology laboratories, the half-life of the drugs in overdose is so short that it is of no clinical value to measure this routinely.

Liver and renal function tests may become abnormal and acute renal failure and gastrointestinal bleeding have been described rarely. Therefore electrolytes, liver function tests and a full blood count should be checked in large ingestions.

Warning! Think about the possibility of a NSAID overdose in any young patient presenting with fits.

Supportive care
The half-lives of the drugs are short (several hours) and the drugs are highly protein bound, so elimination methods are not needed. Features of toxicity are unlikely to develop for the first time later than 4 hours after the overdose was taken. Give 50 g activated charcoal for an adult, or 1 mg/kg for a child, if >100 mg/kg body weight of ibuprofen or more than 10 tablets of other NSAIDs have been taken in the last 1 hour. Beyond 1 hour, charcoal is unlikely to be of benefit (p. 10). Maintain the airway and assist ventilation if necessary. Treat non-self-limiting seizures with diazepam i.v. (0.1–0.2 mg/kg). Oral H_2 blockers (e.g. ranitidine 300 mg/day orally) may ease symptoms of gastrointestinal irritation.

Further reading
Menzies DG, Conn AG, Williamson IJ. Fulminant hyperkalaemia and multiple complications following ibuprofen overdose. Med Tox Adver Drug Exp 1989; 4: 468–471.

Smolinske SC, Hall AH, Vandenberg SA. Toxic effects of nonsteroidal anti-inflammatory drugs in overdose. Drug Safety 1990; 5: 252–274.

Hall AH, Smolinske SC, Stover B. Ibuprofen overdose in adults. Clin Toxicol 1992; 30: 23–37.

OPIOIDS: HEROIN, MORPHINE, METHADONE, CODEINE, PETHIDINE, DIHYDROCODEINE, DEXTROPROPOXYPHENE

The hallmarks of opioid analgesic poisoning are:

- Depressed respiration
- Pin-point or small pupils
- Depressed consciousness level
- Signs of intravenous drug abuse (e.g. needle track marks).

Respiratory arrest, systemic hypotension, non-cardiogenic pulmonary oedema and hypothermia indicate severe poisoning. Convulsions are common in children. Death occurs by respiratory arrest or from aspiration of gastric contents.

Dextropropoxyphene (the opioid in co-proxamol) poisoning may also result in cardiac conduction effects, particularly QRS prolongation, ventricular arrhythmias and heart block due to its membrane stabilising activity.

Symptoms can be prolonged for up to 24–48 hours, particularly after ingestion of methadone which has a long half-life.

Steps should be taken to ensure a clear airway and support respiration if necessary. The need for endotracheal intubation can often be avoided by prompt administration of adequate doses of naloxone, the opioid antagonist.

> Warning! Opioid tablets are frequently co-formulated with paracetamol – be careful not to miss the paracetamol overdose.

Essential laboratory investigations

Oxygen saturation and arterial blood gases demonstrate the adequacy of ventilation in those whose respiration has been compromised.

Qualitative screening of the urine (e.g. *Syva* EMIT assay) is an effective way to confirm recent use. Routine screens may, however, not detect fentanyl derivatives, tramadol and other synthetic opioids. Occasionally, measuring opioids and their metabolites in blood is required for medico-legal purposes, particularly where there is a fatality or a child is poisoned. In circumstances such as these urine and serum should be saved for later analysis.

Supportive care

Maintain an open airway and assist ventilation if necessary. Give supplemental high flow oxygen. Treat coma (p. 16), fits (p. 23) and hypotension (p. 16) if they occur.

Give activated charcoal (50 g in adults, 1 g/kg in children) if a patient presents within 1 hour of ingestion of a substantial amount of opioids (ensure that the airway is protected).

Non-cardiogenic pulmonary oedema in severe cases often fails to respond to loop diuretics – **CPAP and/or PEEP** may be required in these cases.

i.v. sodium bicarbonate (p. 14) may be effective for QRS interval prolongation or hypotension associated with dextropropoxyphene poisoning.

Owing to the large volume of distribution of opioids and the availability of an effective antidote, enhanced elimination procedures are not used.

Specific measures

Naloxone is a specific opioid antagonist, which reverses the above features of opioid toxicity. Use Naloxone 0.8–2 mg intravenously for an adult as bolus doses (0.01 mg/kg for a child). This dose should be repeated every 2 minutes as necessary until the level of consciousness and respiratory rate increase (and the pupils dilate). A total dose of as much as 10–20 mg may be required in some cases! Try not to overdo antidote administration, however, as it can precipitate a withdrawal reaction (characterised by gastrointestinal effects, sweating and fits). Make the naloxone up in at least a 5 ml syringe and titrate repeat bolus doses according to response. Aim for GCS 13–14 (not 15 and leaving your department!). If patients are insistent on leaving, an i.m. dose of 1.2 mg is helpful to delay absorption of the antidote and prevent a respiratory arrest occurring as soon as the i.v. dose of naloxone has worn off.

After the initial i.v. bolus, an infusion of naloxone may be needed, because the half-life of the antidote is much shorter than the half-life of most opioids. Infusion of two-thirds of the bolus dose initially required to wake the patient should be given each hour – this can be given diluted in saline 0.9%. Patients must be carefully observed for recurrence of coma and respiratory depression, usually for at least 18–24 hours. It is particularly important that patients are observed for recurrence of CNS depression for at least 4–6 hours after the last dose of naloxone is given.

Naloxone has been reported to cause pulmonary oedema and ventricular arrhythmias but they do not occur frequently enough to outweigh its use.

Warning! Failure to respond to naloxone may indicate use of inadequate doses or the wrong diagnosis – several mgs may be required.
The half-life of the drug is always longer than that of naloxone, and therefore repeated administration or an infusion of naloxone is almost always required. Administration of naloxone to addicts may cause withdrawal characterised by abdominal cramps, diarrhoea, piloerection and vasoconstriction. This is usually short-lived.

Further reading

Goldfrank L, Weisman RS, Errick JK. A dosing nomogram for continuous infusion of intravenous naloxone. Ann Emerg Med 1986; 15: 566–570.

Watson WA. Opioid toxicity recurrence after an initial response to naloxone. Clin Toxicol 1998; 36: 11–17.

TABLE 2.4   Common adult preparations containing paracetamol

Product	Content per tablet
Paracetamol 500 mg	Paracetamol 500 mg
Co-codamol 8/500	Codeine phosphate 8 mg; paracetamol 500 mg
Co-codamol 30/500	Codeine phosphate 30 mg; paracetamol 500 mg
Co-proxamol	Dextropropoxyphene 32.5 mg; paracetamol 325 mg
Co-dydramol	Dihydrocodeine 10 mg; paracetamol 500 mg

PARACETAMOL (ACETAMINOPHEN)

Paracetamol is the commonest drug taken in overdose in the UK. 150 mg/kg paracetamol has been recognised as a hepatotoxic dose for most people and should be used as a threshold to guide therapy such as activated charcoal and gastric lavage (see flowcharts 2.2a and 2.2b). Chronic alcohol ingestion (>14 units/week for women, >21 units/week for men) has been reported to reduce the ceiling of toxicity of paracetamol and 75 mg/kg is potentially toxic in these groups. In addition, adolescents with eating disorders or others with glutathione depletion may be at increased risk, as may patients who are taking enzyme-inducing drugs such as phenytoin, carbamazepine, phenobarbitone, rifampicin. Paradoxically, acute ingestion with ethanol reduces the toxicity of paracetamol, but the 150 mg/kg rule to guide treatment should still be used.

It is important to err on the side of treating any patient with N-acetylcysteine if the blood concentration lies near but just below the treatment line because stated timing of the overdose may be inaccurate and other agents may slow gastric emptying, e.g. co-ingestion of opioid drugs.

Paracetamol poisoning is deceptive, as in the early phases it is common for the patient to remain asymptomatic, although there may be nausea and vomiting. Liver damage (with abdominal pain or tenderness) or rarely renal damage may begin to appear from 24 hours after ingestion. Renal failure occurs in only a small proportion of patients, usually, but not always, those with severe liver damage and hepatic failure. Renal angle pain or tenderness may warn of incipient renal failure. Loss of consciousness indicates that something else has been taken in addition to paracetamol (often an opioid). The key clinical action is to start the antidote (N-acetylcysteine) as early as possible and if it is given within 12 hours, it provides complete protection against liver injury and renal failure. If there is doubt about whether to treat, it is important to err on the side of giving N-acetylcysteine. Treatment flowcharts 2.2a and 2.2b provide a guide to management – if in any doubt, advice is always available from a centre of the National Poisons Information Service.

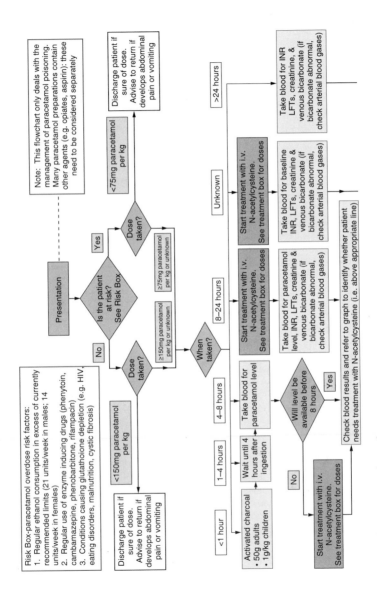

Fig. 2.2a Single paracetamol overdose

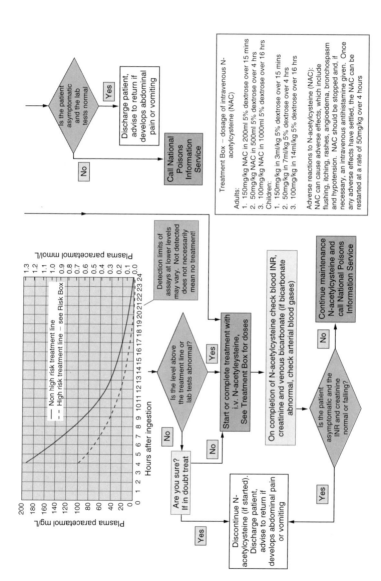

Fig. 2.2a (Cont.)

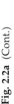

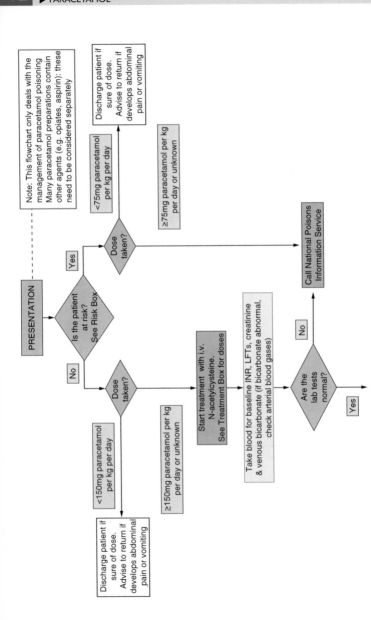

Fig. 2.2b Staggered paracetamol overdose

Risk Box – paracetamol overdose risk factors:
1. Regular ethanol consumption in excess of currently recommended limits (21 units/week in males; 14 units/week in females)
2. Regular use of enzyme inducing drugs (phenytoin, carbamazepine, phenobarbitone, rifampacin)
3. Conditions causing glutathione depletion (e.g. HIV, eating disorders, malnutrition, cystic fibrosis)

Treatment Box – Dosage of Intravenous N-acetylcysteine (NAC)

Adults:
1. 150mg/kg NAC in 200ml 5% dextrose over 15 mins
2. 50mg/kg NAC in 500ml 5% dextrose over 4 hrs
3. 100mg/kg NAC in 1000ml 5% dextrose over 16 hrs
Children:
1. 150mg/kg in 3ml/kg 5% dextrose over 15 mins
2. 50mg/kg 7ml/kg 5% dextrose over 4 hrs
3. 100mg/kg in 14ml/kg 5% dextrose over 16 hrs

Adverse reactions to N-acetylcysteine (NAC):
NAC can cause adverse effects, which include flushing, itching, rashes, angioedema, bronchospasm and hypotension. NAC should be stopped and, if necessary, an intravenous antihistamine given. Once any adverse effects have settled, the NAC can be restarted at a rate of 50mg/kg over 4 hrs.

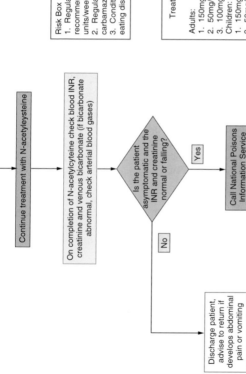

Continue treatment with N-acetyleysteine

On completion of N-acetylcyteine check blood INR, creatinine and venous bicarbonate (if bicarbonate abnormal, check arterial blood gases)

Is the patient asymptomatic and the INR and creatinine normal or falling?

Yes

No

Call National Poisons Information Service

Discharge patient, advise to return if develops abdominal pain or vomiting

Fig. 2.2b (Cont.)

> Warning! Beware 'at risk' groups including those with induced enzymes and those with glutathione depletion – they need treatment at lower plasma paracetamol levels.
> Beware of the detection limit of the paracetamol assay. This becomes important beyond 15 hours after ingestion when undetectable levels do not necessarily indicate that no treatment is required.
> Beware the patient with abdominal pain and hidden paracetamol overdose.

Late paracetamol poisoning

It is important that patients who present after 24 hours with poisoning due to paracetamol receive meticulous supportive care, including monitoring of acid-base status, prothrombin ratio (PTR) and creatinine. Such patients should usually receive i.v. N-acetylcysteine straight away and then be discussed with a poisons centre or a liver transplant unit. Transplant criteria include: arterial blood pH <7.3 after resuscitation or PT >100 seconds and serum creatinine >300 μmol/L in patients with Grade III or IV encephalopathy, and it is important to have such results available when making the call. Because of the importance of PTR in determining severity and prognosis, it is important that vitamin K or fresh frozen plasma are *not* given to patients, unless they are actively bleeding.

If hepatic damage is extensive, hepatic failure ensues on the fourth or fifth day (though it can be quicker) with encephalopathy, hypoglycaemia and coagulopathy. Sepsis may prevail and cerebral oedema is a common mode of death unless successful liver transplantation takes place.

Two-stage or staggered overdoses

The best solution in two-stage overdoses, i.e. doses taken at two time points, is to interpret the plasma paracetamol concentration as if it were the result of all the drug having been ingested at the time of first overdose. This errs on the safe side in treating with N-acetylcysteine.

If multiple overdoses have been taken over one or more days, a plasma paracetamol concentration cannot be used to guide the need for treatment and it is wise to treat anyone with N-acetylcysteine who has ingested more than 150 mg paracetamol/kg body weight/day (>75 mg/kg/day for at risk groups).

Chronic toxicity

Has been reported after daily consumption of high therapeutic doses of paracetamol. If >150 mg/kg/day have been taken (>75 mg/kg/day for at risk groups), treatment with N-acetylcysteine is advised.

Paracetamol poisoning in children

Most paracetamol overdoses in young children involve paediatric formulations, which limit the amount ingested. As a result it is very unusual to get serious poisoning in children from such products. Although children may be less susceptible to paracetamol toxicity than adults, the same treatment applies.

TABLE 2.5   Toxic paracetamol doses (150 mg/kg) in children

Body weight (kg)	Amount of paracetamol that would be toxic	Equivalent to
10	1 500 mg	12 spoons of syrup 125 mg/5 ml
20	3 000 mg	12 spoons of syrup 250 mg/5 ml
30	4 500 mg	18 spoons of syrup 250 mg/5 ml
40	6 000 mg	12 × 500 mg tablets
50	7 500 mg	15 × 500 mg tablets

NB: 75 mg/kg should be used as the toxic dose for children on enzyme-inducing drugs (e.g. phenytoin, carbamazepine, rifampicin) and those who are malnourished (e.g. cystic fibrosis, cyanotic congenital heart disease).

Paracetamol overdose in pregnancy
Paracetamol is not teratogenic, though untreated paracetamol poisoning may cause hepatotoxicity to mother and fetus. The mother should be treated using standard treatment protocols (see flowcharts 2.2a and 2.2b).

Essential laboratory investigations (see flowcharts 2.2a and 2.2b)
The plasma paracetamol concentration is used to guide the need for antidote (N-acetylcysteine) administration. A blood sample should not be taken for plasma paracetamol estimation before 4 hours have elapsed since the overdose (because it is not interpretable until then).

Blood should be taken for paracetamol estimation whenever an unconscious patient is admitted and poisoning by paracetamol cannot be ruled out. In this respect beware of opioid/paracetamol combinations such as co-proxamol (dextropropoxyphene and paracetamol). Occasionally, very high plasma paracetamol concentrations are seen – this can be associated with a metabolic (lactic) acidosis.

The most sensitive marker of prognosis in paracetamol poisoning is the prothrombin ratio (PTR) or INR. This often starts to increase within 24–36 hours of the overdose and tends to peak at 48–72 hours. Once the PTR starts to improve, this is a sign that hepatotoxicity is starting to improve and the patient will not go on to develop fulminant hepatic failure. Approximately 50% of patients who have a prothrombin time of 36 seconds at 36 hours will go on to develop fulminant hepatic failure.

Plasma alanine and aspartate aminotranferases (ALT and AST) may begin to rise as early as 12 hours but peaks do not usually occur until 72–96 hours after the overdose. ASTs or ALTs of 12 000 IU/L are not uncommon. A plasma ALT of >5 000 IU/L is very suggestive of a diagnosis of paracetamol poisoning. Serum bilirubin tends to peak after the aminotransferases and this should not lead to unnecessary concern in patients whose PTR is falling.

Hypoglycaemia and metabolic acidosis are common in paracetamol poisoning. Pancreatitis with raised serum amylase has also been reported.

Use of intravenous N-acetylcysteine

● 150 mg/kg body weight in 200 ml 5% dextrose for 15 minutes

  followed by

● 50 mg/kg in 500 ml 5% dextrose over 4 hours

  followed by

● 100 mg/kg in 1000 ml 5% dextrose over 16 hours.

Adverse reactions to intravenous N-acetylcysteine have been reported in up to 5% of patients and are most likely to occur during the first hour when the plasma concentrations are at their highest. These 'anaphylactoid' reactions include nausea, vomiting, flushing, urticaria and pruritus. Such reactions settle with stopping the infusion for half an hour and if necessary giving an oral or intravenous antihistamine and restarting at the 50 mg/kg over 4 hour infusion. In view of the risk of anaphylactoid reactions, there has been a vogue to commence N-acetylcysteine infusions at a slower rate than 150 mg/kg over 15 minutes, but such protocols do not yet have proven efficacy. More severe reactions include bronchospasm, angio-oedema and systemic hypotension and these require cessation of N-acetylcysteine and administration of subcutaneous adrenaline. If a patient has developed a true anaphylactic reaction to N-acetylcysteine, an alternative antidote can be used. This is oral methionine at a dose of 2.5 g orally every 4 hours to a total dose of 10 g. However methionine is not as good as N-acetylcysteine in late paracetamol poisoning and has limited efficacy at greater than 8 hours after ingestion.

Further reading

Prescott LF, Illingworth RN, Critchley JA, Proudfoot AT. Intravenous N-acetylcysteine: the treatment of choice for paracetamol poisoning. BMJ 1979; 2: 1097–1100.

Dawson AH, Henry DA, McEwen J. Adverse reactions to N-acetylcysteine during treatment for paracetamol poisoning. Med J Aust 1989; 150: 1329–1331.

Dargan PI, Wallace C, Jones AL. A flowchart for management of paracetamol poisoning. J Accid Emerg Med (in press).

O'Grady JG, Alexander GJM, Hayllar KM, Williams R. Early indicators of poor prognosis in fulminant hepatic failure. Gastroenterol 1989; 97: 439–445.

Keays R, Harrison PM, Wendon JA, Forbes A, Gove C, Alexander GJM. Intravenous acetylcysteine in paracetamol induced fulminant hepatic failure: a prospective controlled trial. BMJ 1991; 303: 1026–1029.

Jones AL, Prescott LF. Unusual complications of paracetamol poisoning. Q J Med 1997; 90: 161–168.

Paracetamol Wallchart 1999, Paracetamol Information Centre, London.

PHENOTHIAZINES

Phenothiazines are antipsychotic agents used in the treatment of schizophrenia. They include chlorpromazine, methotrimeprazine, pericyazine, pipothiazine, thioridazine, fluphenazine, perphenazine, prochlorperazine and trifluoperazine. Features of overdose with phenothiazines include drowsiness, hypotension and hypothermia. Extrapyramidal effects are also common including tremor, rigidity and acute dystonic reactions. Rarely QRS and QT_c prolongation, arrhythmias and convulsions may develop.

Activated charcoal should be given, and gastric lavage considered, for patients who have taken a large overdose and present within 1 hour of ingestion. Extrapyramidal symptoms should be treated with procyclidine (adults: 5–10 mg i.v. or i.m. to a maximum of 20 mg/24 hours; children: <2 years 0.5–2 mg, >2 years 2–5 mg, >10 years 5–10 mg i.m. or i.v., repeated after 20 minutes if necessary) or benztropine (adults: 1–2 mg i.m. or i.v. repeated as required; children: 20 μg/kg/dose i.m., i.v. or p.o.). All patients should be observed for 4 to 6 hours after ingestion – patients who remain symptomatic at this stage should be observed for 24 hours post-ingestion with cardiac monitoring. Ventricular arrhythmias, if they occur, should be treated with cardioversion, phenytoin or lignocaine. Class Ia antiarrhythmics are contraindicated (quinidine, disopyramide, procainamide). In severe cases, or if torsade de pointes develops, arrhythmias may be unresponsive to both drug therapy and cardioversion, and transvenous pacing is necessary (pp. 19, 20).

PHENYTOIN

Phenytoin is widely used for the control of tonic–clonic and psychomotor seizures.

Clinical features

In overdose, the absorption of phenytoin from the gastrointestinal tract may be delayed and continue for as long as 60 hours, and has been reported up to 230 hours. The minimum half-life in overdosage appears to be 7 hours, but can be delayed up to 60 hours.

Nausea and vomiting occur with 1–2 hours of a substantial ingestion of phenytoin. As concentrations of the drug increase, spontaneous horizontal nystagmus is seen. Later, vertical nystagmus, dysarthria, drowsiness, ataxia and coarse tremor become apparent. Hyperreflexia, hyporeflexia, opisthotonus and seizures can be seen with high drug concentrations. Cerebellar signs usually improve as serum concentrations fall, but this may take up to 5 days. Cardiovascular toxicity is rare unless the overdose has been given i.v. in which case it is probably due to the propylene glycol diluent. Rarely, bradycardia, atrioventricular block, hypotension and asystole have been seen. Rare features of phenytoin overdose include hepatocellular damage, hyperglycaemia and hypernatraemia.

> **Warning!** Horizontal nystagmus is the *sine qua non* of phenytoin toxicity.
> Coma and respiratory depression are so unusual with phenyton intoxication that, if
> present, they point to another cause, e.g. head injury or another drug in overdose.

Essential investigations

Peak plasma concentrations may not be attained for 24–48 hours. Phenytoin toxicity is not normally seen with plasma concentrations of less than 15 mg/L (60 mmol/L). Nystagmus occurs with concentrations of at least 20 mg/L (80 mmol/L) and ataxia at levels of 30–40 mg/L (120–160 mmol/L). Deaths are usually associated with plasma concentrations above 90 mg/L (360 mmol/L).

Supportive care

Most patients require nothing more than supportive measures. Asymptomatic patients with nystagmus should be observed for 6 hours; patients with nystagmus and impaired consciousness should be observed for 24 hours. Activated charcoal should be given (and gastric lavage should be considered) if a patient presents within 1 hour of a significant overdose (p. 10). Multiple-dose activated charcoal can also be given (p. 13), as it may increase phenytoin elimination, but there is no data to confirm whether this is of clinical benefit. Seizures should be treated with diazepam 0.1–0.2 mg/kg i.v. to a maximum of 30 mg in an adult.

Specific measures

Phenytoin is highly protein bound and therefore forced diuresis, peritoneal dialysis, plasmapheresis and haemodialysis are not of value.

Charcoal haemoperfusion has been used in severe poisoning but is of questionable value and is rarely necessary in lone phenytoin poisoning.

Further reading

Jones AL, Proudfoot AT. Features and management of poisoning with modern drugs used to treat epilepsy. Q J Med 1998; 91: 325–332.

QUININE

Quinine salts are used in the treatment of malaria and nocturnal cramps. Quinine has also been used to cut street heroin. The average fatal dose in an adult is 8 g although deaths have been reported from as little as 1.5 g in an adult and 900 mg in a child. Quinine has toxic effects on the retina that can result in blindness. This effect is partly due to retinal vasoconstriction, but quinine also has a direct toxic effect on retinal photoreceptor cells.

Clinical features

The onset of effects is rapid and early features include nausea, vomiting, tinnitus, deafness, headache and tremor. In large overdoses ataxia, drowsiness, coma, respiratory depression, haemolysis, cardiac effects and retinal toxicity can occur. Cardiac effects include hypotension, ECG changes (prolongation of the QRS and QT_c intervals, AV block) and arrhythmias (VT, torsade de pointes and VF). Retinal toxicity usually occurs 6–10 hours after ingestion, initially with blurred vision and impaired colour perception. This can progress to constriction of the visual fields, scotomata and complete blindness. The pupils become dilated and unresponsive to light and fundoscopy shows retinal artery spasm progressing to disc pallor and retinal oedema. Visual loss can be permanent.

Essential investigations

All patients should have a 12-lead ECG and blood should be taken for U&Es and glucose because quinine can cause hypokalaemia and hypoglycaemia.

Supportive care

Maintenance of the airway, breathing and ventilation is critical. Gastric lavage should be considered if a patient presents within 1 hour of ingestion of >15 mg/kg of quinine. Multiple-dose activated charcoal (50 g 4-hourly in an adult, 1 g/kg body weight 4-hourly in a child) should be given to all patients who have ingested >15 mg/kg quinine. All patients should be put on a cardiac monitor for at least 6 hours.

Specific measures

Visual effects of quinine are largely untreatable. In the past many measures were advocated, e.g. stellate ganglion block, retrobulbar injections, or vasodilators including nitrates. However these make little difference to outcome and we would not advocate their routine use.

Cardiotoxicity: treat hypotension with i.v. fluid replacement. Inotropes may also be necessary. Sodium bicarbonate i.v. is the treatment of choice for arrhythmias and should also be used in patients with widened QRS and QT_c intervals (dose: 1–2 ml/kg 8.4% sodium bicarbonate, repeated if necessary, aiming for a pH of 7.45–7.5). The treatment of choice for VT and torsade de pointes is overdrive pacing (p. 20). All antiarrhythmic drugs are potentially arrhythmogenic and should therefore be avoided. Class I agents in particular are contraindicated and lignocaine should not be used because it may precipitate convulsions (p. 18).

Haemodialysis and haemoperfusion are ineffective in quinine poisoning and urinary acidification is not advised because although it may increase renal excretion slightly, it worsens cardiotoxicity.

RIFAMPICIN

This is an antituberculous drug. It is well absorbed orally with a half-life of 4–5 hours after ingestion. The half-life may be prolonged in slow acetylators and those with liver disease. In therapeutic doses, rifampicin has been associated with hepatitis.

Rifampicin in overdose can produce a characteristic orange staining of tissues and urine. Peculiarly, the skin colour can be partly removed by scrubbing or vigorous washing, a feature unique to rifampicin.

Overdose is characterised by gastrointestinal effects such as nausea and vomiting, flushing, pulmonary oedema and confusion. Some patients have died from pulmonary oedema. Death is commoner in those with underlying liver disorders.

Gastric lavage can be undertaken if the patient presents within 1 hour of ingestion. Because rifampicin undergoes enterohepatic circulation, multiple-dose activated charcoal (p. 13) may increase clearance and is recommended. Rifampicin is not well cleared by haemodialysis or haemoperfusion and these are not recommended.

> Warning! Rifampicin is often taken together with isoniazid (for which the antidote is pyridoxine) in overdose.

RISPERIDONE

This is an antipsychotic drug used in the treatment of schizophrenia. Few overdoses have been reported. Features of overdose include drowsiness, hallucinations, tachycardia, prolonged QRS and QT_c intervals and extrapyramidal effects including tremor, rigidity and acute dystonic reactions. Activated charcoal should be given (and gastric lavage considered) for ingestion of >100 mg by an adult within the last 1 hour. Observation and ECG monitoring should be carried out for a minimum of 12 hours post-ingestion.

Extrapyramidal symptoms should be treated with procyclidine (adults: 5–10 mg i.v. or i.m. to a maximum of 20 mg/24 hours; children: <2 years 0.5–2 mg, >2 years 2–5 mg, >10 years 5–10 mg i.m. or i.v., repeated after 20 minutes if necessary) or benztropine (adults: 1–2 mg i.m. or i.v. repeated as required; children: 20 μg/kg/dose i.m., i.v. or p.o.). Ventricular arrhythmias, if they occur, should be treated with cardioversion, phenytoin or lignocaine. Class Ia antiarrhythmics are contraindicated (quinidine, disopyramide, procainamide). In severe cases, or if torsade de pointes develops, arrhythmias may be unresponsive to both drug therapy and cardioversion, and transvenous pacing is necessary (p. 20).

SALICYLATES (ASPIRIN)

Salicylate or aspirin poisoning is much less common than 20 years ago but because of this doctors may fail to recognise its severity or treat such patients optimally.

Clinical features

More than 150, 250 and 500 mg/kg body weight produces mild, moderate and severe (potentially fatal) poisoning respectively and management of poisoning is shown in the flowchart 2.3. Although overdose with aspirin tablets is the commonest cause, salicylate poisoning can also occur with ingestion of other salicylates such as oil of wintergreen or when salicylic ointment (e.g. verruca remover) is applied extensively to skin or swallowed.

Salicylate overdose commonly produces nausea, vomiting, tinnitus and deafness. Direct stimulation of the respiratory centre produces hyperventilation. This is more common in adults, who often have a respiratory alkalosis at presentation. Children more commonly develop a metabolic acidosis. Peripheral vasodilation with bounding pulses and profuse sweating occurs in moderately severe poisoning. Hypoglycaemia is relatively common in children but rare in adults. Petechiae and subconjunctival haemorrhages can occur and are due to reduced platelet aggregation and are self-limiting.

Signs of serious salicylate poisoning include metabolic acidosis, renal failure and CNS effects such as agitation, confusion, coma and fits. Rarely, hyperpyrexia, pulmonary oedema and cerebral oedema occur. Death is by CNS depression and cardiovascular collapse. The development of a metabolic acidosis is a bad prognostic sign, not least because acidosis results in increased salicylate transfer across the blood–brain barrier.

Warning! Beware the patient with CNS features or acidosis; these indicate severe poisoning and the need for early haemodialysis.
Young children and the elderly are at greatest risk from salicylate poisoning.

Essential laboratory investigations (see flowchart 2.3)
It is important to measure a plasma salicylate concentration in all but the most trivial overdose and this should be done on an urgent basis. However, this should be delayed in patients who present early until 4 hours after ingestion, because the result is not interpretable until this stage. The salicylate level is not an absolute guide to toxicity and needs to be interpreted together with clinical features and the acid–base status.

Salicylates tend to form concretions within the stomach which delay absorption and so it is wise to recheck a plasma salicylate concentration 3–4 hours after the first sample, to catch the salicylate peak blood concentration. Unlike the situation with paracetamol poisoning, there is no evidence for indiscriminate use of plasma salicylate estimations in every unconscious patient.

Acid–base disturbances are common in salicylate poisoning and its accurate assessment demands arterial blood gas sampling. Respiratory stimulation causes hyperventilation and a consequent respiratory alkalosis. At the same time (often) uncoupling of oxidative phosphorylation and interruption of glucose and fatty acid metabolism by salicylates causes a lactic acidosis and production of other organic acids, resulting in a metabolic acidosis. Children are more likely to have a metabolic acidosis whereas adults tend to show a mixed respiratory alkalosis and metabolic acidosis. Acidosis leads to greater movement of salicylate across the blood–brain barrier and should be avoided. Serial ABGs are needed in moderate–severe poisoning (see p. 7 for interpretation of blood gases).

Fluid balance and electrolytes also need to be carefully monitored in patients with moderate–severe salicylate poisoning.

Supportive care (see flowchart 2.3)
Treat metabolic acidosis with intravenous sodium bicarbonate, 50 ml of 8.4% sodium bicarbonate i.v. titrated to a pH of 7.4. Replace fluid loss from

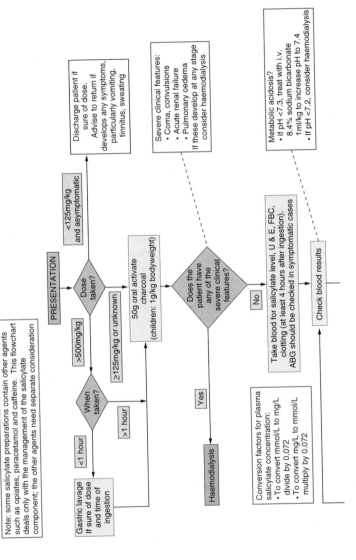

Fig. 2.3 Salicylate overdose

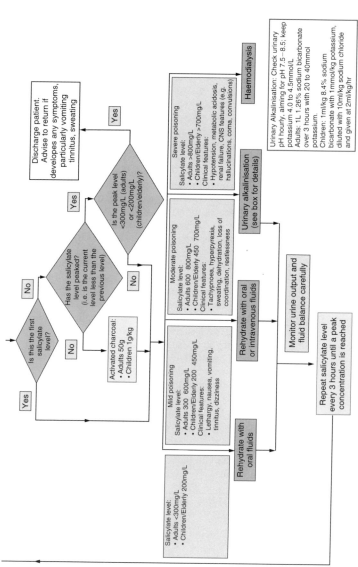

Fig. 2.3 (Cont.)

vomiting and sweating (patients are often very dehydrated) with i.v. fluids. However, be careful not to fluid overload these patients as they have increased risk of pulmonary oedema – in the elderly or those with cardiac disease a central line is often necessary to guide fluid management.

For gastric decontamination in salicylate overdose see the flowchart. The use of multiple-dose activated charcoal (MDAC) in salicylate poisoning is controversial. We advocate the use of MDAC until the salicylate level has peaked.

Specific measures

Urinary alkalinisation is indicated for patients with salicylate concentrations 600–800 mg/L in adults and 450–700 mg/L in children and the elderly. 1 L of sodium bicarbonate 1.26% is given intravenously over 3 hours for an adult. Ensure urinary alkalinisation (aiming for a urinary pH 7.5–8.5) is achieved by checking the pH of the urine with indicator paper. Also check plasma potassium, as it is very difficult to produce an alkaline urine if the patient is hypokalaemic and also potassium can fall precipitously once adequate urinary alkalinisation commences and so it is wise to add 20–40 mmol potassium to each litre of i.v. fluid administered. Alkalosis is not a contraindication to bicarbonate therapy, as patients have a high base deficit in spite of the elevated serum pH.

Haemodialysis is very effective at removing salicylate and correcting acid–base and fluid balance abnormalities. It should be considered for an acute ingestion resulting in serum concentrations of >800 mg/L in adults and >700 mg/L in children and the elderly. Other indications for haemodialysis in acute salicylate overdose are metabolic acidosis resistant to correction, severe CNS effects such as coma or convulsions, pulmonary oedema and acute renal failure. It is also useful in chronic intoxication for levels greater than 600 mg/L, particularly in a confused elderly patient. Haemoperfusion is also effective, but does not correct acid–base disturbances, and so haemodialysis is the preferred method.

Further reading

Chapman BJ, Proudfoot AT. Adult salicylate poisoning: deaths and outcome in patients with high plasma salicylate concentrations. Q J Med 1989; 72: 699–707.

Dargan PI, Jones AL. Flowchart for the management of salicylate poisoning J Accid Emerg Med (in press).

SELECTIVE SEROTONIN RE-UPTAKE INHIBITORS (SSRIs) OR 5HT DRUGS

Common serotonin uptake inhibitors taken in overdose:

- Citalopram
- Fluoxetine
- Fluvoxamine

- Paroexetine
- Sertraline
- Venlafaxine.

Clinical features

This class of antidepressants does not have the anticholinergic actions of the tricyclic antidepressants (TCAs). In addition they are much less cardiotoxic and cause fewer deaths in overdose than TCAs. Drowsiness and sinus tachycardia are the most common effects in overdose, but the extent is much less than in TCA poisoning. Citalopram has caused a nodal rhythm with QT and QRS prolongation and fluoxetine may cause minor ST-T wave changes. Nausea and diarrhoea are also common. Seizures can occur but are more common after venlafaxine overdose. Dizziness, dilated pupils, tremor, agitation, dry mouth, junctional bradycardia and hypertension have also been reported.

The serotonin syndrome (p. 25) can be caused by administration of two or more agents that increase serotonin availability in the CNS, such as SSRIs and MAOIs.

Essential investigations

None, unless level of consciousness is significantly impaired.

Warning! Check the patient has indeed taken an SSRI or 5HT drug and not a tricyclic antidepressant. QRS prolongation suggests a tricyclic antidepressant overdose.
Check if there is an interaction with other SSRIs or MAOIs which may cause a serotonin syndrome.

Supportive care

Supportive and symptomatic measures are all that are required. Give activated charcoal if an adult has ingested more than 10 tablets within the last 1 hour. Observation for 6 hours is recommended, with cardiac monitoring in symptomatic cases. Rarely coma, hypotension and fits will require treatment (pp. 16, 23).

Further reading

Borys DJ, Setzer SC, Ling LJ et al. The effects of fluoxetine in the overdose patient. Clin Toxicol 1990; 28: 331–340.

Neuvonen PJ, Pohjola-Sintonene S, Tacke U, Vuori E. Five fatal cases of serotonin syndrome after moclobemide-citalopram or moclobemide-clomipramine overdose. Lancet 1993; 342: 1419.

Personne M, Sjoberg G, Persson H. Citalopram overdose – review of cases treated in Swedish hospitals. Clin Toxicol 1997; 35: 237–240.

Sternbach H. The serotonin syndrome. Am J Psychiatry 1991; 148: 705–713.

Phillips S, Brent J, Kulig K, Heiligensten J, Birkett M. Fluoxetine versus tricyclic antidepressants: A prospective multicenter study of antidepressant drug overdoses. J Emerg Med 1997; 15: 439–445.

SILDENAFIL (VIAGRA)

Sildenafil is used in the treatment of impotence. There have been few overdoses reported. Clinical effects are likely to include headache, flushing, dizziness and altered vision. Ventricular arrhythmias and myocardial infarction have been recorded in therapeutic use. Vasodilation and severe hypotension can occur if sildenafil is taken together with nitrates or nitrites. Activated charcoal should be given if an adult presents within 1 hour of ingestion of more than 800 mg of sildenafil (or for any amount in a child). Patients should be observed with ECG monitoring for 4 hours after ingestion.

SULPHONYLUREAS: see ANTIDIABETIC AGENTS

SULPIRIDE

Sulpiride is an antipsychotic used in the treatment of schizophrenia. It is generally of relatively low toxicity in overdose. The fatal dose in adults is not known, but survival after ingestion of 16 grams has been reported.

Clinical features seen after overdose include restlessness, drowsiness, agitation and extrapyramidal effects, and more rarely coma and hypotension in massive overdose. Onset of symptoms is within 1–2 hours of overdose and effects may continue for up to 24–48 hours. Patients should be observed for at least 6 hours, and most patients will have only mild effects following overdose. If the patient is severely affected (e.g. intractable hypotension) enhanced elimination with urinary alkalinisation can be considered, although there is no evidence of the efficacy of this procedure. Sulpiride is less than 40% protein bound and has a relatively low volume of distribution. In critically ill cases, therefore, haemodialysis may be considered although again there is no evidence for its efficacy.

THEOPHYLLINE

Acute theophylline poisoning is potentially very serious and severe poisoning carries a high mortality. Severe toxicity is expected with ingestion of 3 g in adults and 40 mg/kg in children. Theophylline is most commonly used orally in sustained-release preparations. Overdosage with these products undergoes delayed absorption which can result in delayed onset of toxicity, as late as 12–24 hours.

Clinical features of acute overdose
Tachycardia is extremely common in theophylline poisoning. Continuing or increasing tachycardia and the development of ectopic beats are signs of

worsening toxicity. Blood pressure may be raised initially but falls later. Supraventricular tachycardia and ventricular ectopics may precede ventricular arrhythmias.

Nausea, intractable vomiting and diarrhoea are very common. Haematemesis can occur and may be severe.

CNS stimulation with restlessness, hyperactivity and anxiety are common. Dilation of the pupils, tremor, convulsions and hyperventilation are also common. Hypertonia, hyperreflexia and erratic movements of the limbs may occur. Rhabdomyolysis, leucocytosis and hyperpyrexia may also be features. Acute renal failure has been reported.

Metabolic effects include marked hypokalaemia, hypophosphataemia, hypomagnesaemia, hyperglycaemia and metabolic acidosis.

The following system has been proposed for grading severity of theophylline intoxication (Table 2.6).

TABLE 2.6   Severity of theophylline intoxication

Severity grade	Clinical features
1	Vomiting, abdominal pain, diarrhoea, anxiety, tremor, sinus tachycardia >120 beats per minute, plasma potassium <3.5 mmol/L but >2.5 mmol/L.
2	Haematemesis, disorientation, supraventricular tachycardias, frequent ectopics, mean arterial blood pressure at least 60 mmHg but responsive to standard therapy, plasma potassium <2.5 mmol/L, arterial pH <7.2 or >7.6 (hydrogen ion concentration <25 or >63 nmol/L), rhabdomyolysis.
3	Non-repetitive seizure, sustained VT, mean arterial blood pressure <60 mmHg and unresponsive to standard therapy.
4	Recurrent seizures, VF, cardiac arrest.

Essential laboratory investigations for acute overdose

Checking the plasma potassium concentration frequently is essential as hypokalaemia is a potentially life-threatening consequence of theophylline overdosage. In potentially significant poisoning (e.g. ingestion of >20 mg/kg body weight) an arterial blood gas is of value as initial phases of hyperventilation can lead to respiratory alkalosis but as poisoning becomes more severe, metabolic acidosis predominates. The blood glucose should be checked, as hyperglycaemia is common.

Therapeutic plasma concentrations of theophylline do not generally exceed 20 mg/L (155 μmol/L). Theophylline concentrations may exceed 200 mg/L in overdosage and the peak concentration may be attained 1–3 hours after overdose of a non-sustained-release preparation but can be delayed for 8–16 hours after overdose of a sustained-release preparation. The plasma half-life is approximately 10 hours in such cases. Whilst measuring plasma theophylline concentrations helps confirm ingestion and may be of value in deciding upon elimination methods, in the vast majority of poisoned patients they do not aid management. Management is most appropriately guided by the severity on the grading scheme, bearing in mind that delayed effects occur in overdoses with sustained-release formulations. Rarely, in severe cases repeated analyses of theophylline concentrations may be required every 4–6 hours. Most patients who die have grade 4 (sometimes grade 3) toxicity with plasma theophylline concentrations above 100 mg/L (770 μmol/L).

> Warning! Beware sustained-release formulations, where an initial low theophylline blood level does not mean serious poisoning will not occur, and serious toxicity may not be apparent until 12–24 hours after ingestion.
> Do not ignore hypokalaemia.
> The combination of coma, convulsions and vomiting is very hazardous.
> Beware, a caffeine overdose will cause a similar clinical picture and will produce falsely elevated theophylline concentrations with many commercial assays.

Chronic poisoning with theophylline

Taking more than the therapeutic daily dose of theophylline is likely to result in toxicity; chronic toxicity may also be precipitated by intercurrent illness or by drug interactions such as use of cimetidine or erythromycin. Patients with symptoms of theophylline poisoning must be carefully evaluated and plasma theophylline levels are useful. If concentrations are less than 20 mg/L (155 μmol/L) a dose reduction should suffice. Patients with plasma concentrations above 20 mg/L should be treated as described below for an acute overdose. Seizures are particularly common in chronic theophylline poisoning, tachycardia is almost invariable, but vomiting may not be as common. The metabolic effects such as hypokalaemia and hyperglycaemia do not seem common.

Supportive care of acute overdose

Protection of the airway and maintenance of adequate ventilation are necessary if consciousness is impaired. The stomach should be emptied if the patient presents within 1 hour of the overdose unless a small (e.g. less than 20 mg/kg body weight) ingestion has taken place, when charcoal alone can be given promptly. Prompt administration of activated charcoal is vital and this can be first given down the washout tube or orally.

Multiple-dose activated charcoal (MDAC) should be given (50 g orally stat and 50 g 4-hourly for an adult, 1 g/kg per dose for a child). Vomiting can be controlled with conventional anti-emetics such as metoclopramide (10–20 mg i.v. for an adult) or ondansetron (8 mg slowly, i.v. for an adult) if vomiting is intractable. Charcoal should be given via nasogastric tube in a ventilated patient.

Undissolved sustained-release tablets may not be removed with even the largest (40 F) gastric tube. **Whole bowel irrigation** (p. 12) should be considered in the event of a substantial overdose of sustained-release tablets. Alternatively, multiple-doses of activated charcoal could be given if WBI is not available.

The **cardiac rhythm** should be monitored continuously. Sinus or supraventricular tachycardias not causing haemodynamic compromise are best left untreated. In non-asthmatic/COPD patients, symptomatic supraventricular tachycardia should be treated with beta-blockers such as propranolol (0.01–0.03 mg/kg i.v.), metoprolol (5–10 mg i.v.) or esmolol (25–50 μg/kg), repeated according to clinical response. Sometimes, surprisingly large doses are required to treat the tachycardia. If the patient is asthmatic/COPD, disopyramide or verapamil can be used cautiously, and in resistant cases esmolol can be considered because of its short half-life and strong β_1 selectivity. Ventricular arrhythmias are treated with DC cardioversion or magnesium chloride infusion. Lignocaine or mexiletine are best avoided as they may exacerbate convulsions.

Closely **monitor the plasma potassium** and recheck frequently, e.g. every 1–2 hours in severely poisoned patients. Correct hypokalaemia (potassium <2.8 mmol/L) cautiously, by adding potassium chloride to infusion fluids. If non-selective beta-blockers such as propranolol have been given to the patient, the metabolic effects will be partially reversed. Beware of the risk of hyperkalaemia during the recovery phase. Hyperglycaemia is usually transient and well tolerated. Do not overcorrect metabolic acidosis, as it will risk worsening of the hypokalaemia.

Convulsions are best controlled with i.v. diazepam (0.1–0.2 mg/kg). If coma, convulsions and vomiting occur together, it is best to paralyse, intubate and ventilate the patient. This has the advantage of allowing rapid correction of hyperventilation and respiratory alkalosis. However, EEG is still required to exclude ongoing electrical convulsive activity.

Specific measures for acute overdose
It is likely that multiple-dose activated charcoal (MDAC) is almost as effective as charcoal haemoperfusion in the management of severe theophylline poisoning. However, if MDAC is not possible (e.g. paralytic ileus), charcoal haemoperfusion should be considered in grade 3 or 4 poisoning, particularly if plasma concentrations exceed 100 mg/L (770 μmol/L). Lower concentrations (e.g. 60–80 mg/L) may necessitate charcoal haemoperfusion in 'at risk groups' such as the elderly or neonates and those with pre-existing ischaemic heart disease, particularly if they are very unwell. Haemoperfusion should be considered in patients with persistent convulsions despite anticonvulsants and/or intubation and ventilation. Haemodialysis is almost as effective as charcoal haemoperfusion and may be used if the latter is not readily available. It would be preferable to start haemodialysis and give multiple-dose activated charcoal to a severely poisoned patient quickly, than wait for charcoal haemoperfusion or an interhospital transfer to be set up.

Further reading

Ehlers SM, Zaske DE, Sawchuk RJ. Massive theophylline overdose: rapid elimination by charcoal hemoperfusion. JAMA 1978; 240: 474–475.

Janss GJ. Acute theophylline overdose treated with whole bowel irrigation. SDJ Med 1990; 43: 7–8.

Sessler CN. Theophylline toxicity: clinical features of 116 cases. Am J Med 1990; 88: 567–576.

Shannon M. Predictors of major toxicity after theophylline overdose. Ann Intern Med 1993; 119: 1161–1167.

THYROXINE

Only a small proportion of patients who ingest large amounts of thyroxine develop any clinical features of hyperthyroidism (confusion, hyperactivity, tachycardia, mydriasis, sweating, loose stool, headache or pyrexia). Symptoms can develop in a few hours if T3 tri-iodothyronine has been taken, and 3–6 days after overdose of T4 (thyroxine) and resolve within the same time course.

Activated charcoal can be given within 1 hour of ingestion if there is concern about potential toxicity developing from either a T3 or T4 overdose. Blood samples can be taken for estimation of free T4 levels but they are difficult to perform, as dilutional methods are not available in most laboratories. However, if T4 is found to be high 6–12 hours post-ingestion, patients should be reviewed on the 4th or 5th day post-ingestion. In the rare event that symptoms are severe, propranolol (40 mg orally for an adult) is the treatment of choice.

TRICYCLIC ANTIDEPRESSANTS

Common tricyclic antidepressants taken in overdose include:

- Amitriptyline
- Amoxapine
- Dothiepin
- Doxepin
- Impiramine
- Lofepramine
- Loxapine
- Trimipramine.

These drugs remain an important cause of poisoning deaths.

Clinical features

Features of tricyclic antidepressant poisoning include anticholinergic effects (warm, dry skin, tachycardia, blurred vision, large dilated pupils, urinary retention and depressed respiratory and conscious level), seizures and arrhythmias. Reflexes are usually brisk with extensor plantars. Ingestion of more than 10 mg/kg body weight is likely to cause significant toxicity. Uncommon features include divergent squint and pulmonary oedema.

Features of severe poisoning include reduced conscious level, cardiac arrhythmias, fits and hypotension due to myocardial depression. ECG abnormalities are common in moderate–severe poisoning, particularly prolongation of the QRS interval. PR interval prolongation can also occur but second and third degree block are rare. Supraventricular and ventricular dysrhythmias occur and may be the cause of sudden death. Development of bradyarrhythmias usually indicates serious poisoning. Metabolic or respiratory acidosis further contributes to cardiotoxicity.

Death from tricyclic antidepressant poisoning can occur within a few hours of admission and may result from ventricular fibrillation, intractable cardiogenic shock or recurrent seizures, often with aspiration.

Essential investigations

Measurement of the plasma level of a tricyclic antidepressant is not readily available and not helpful in the management of an overdose. An ECG should be performed in all but the most trivial cases of tricyclic antidepressant overdose. A QRS interval of >100 msec carries an increased risk of arrhythmias and >160 msec of fits. However, ECG criteria should not be the only indicator used to assess the severity of poisoning. Amoxapine may cause seizures and coma in the absence of QRS widening.

Arterial blood gas analysis should be performed in patients with marked symptoms, particularly decreased level of consciousness, widened QRS or seizures.

Warning! A patient who has just had a fit is at high risk of a cardiac arrhythmia next – i.e. cardiotoxicity and neurotoxicity tend to go together.
Beware of urine retention due to the anticholinergic effects of the drug – check for a palpable bladder, often.
The combination of sinus tachycardia with conduction abnormalities listed above may lead to the mistaken diagnosis of ventricular tachycardia.

Supportive care

Maintenance of the airway, breathing and ventilation is critical. Gastric lavage can be considered if a substantial amount has been ingested (e.g. more than 20–30 mg/kg weight) within 1 hour. However, there is a risk of pushing contents beyond the pylorus and enhancing absorption of the drug. This, combined with a hypoxic struggling patient, makes the risk of arrhythmias high. Do not wash out an unconscious patient, as clearly significant absorption has already taken place. Activated charcoal (50 g for an adult, 1 g/kg for a child) can be given down the nasogastric tube or by mouth if a patient has ingested more than 10 mg/kg within the last 1 hour. Multiple-dose activated charcoal may be given but is of doubtful efficacy; we would advocate a second dose of charcoal after 2 hours in patients with severe toxicity.

If agitation occurs, diazepam is the drug of choice. It is also the drug of choice for treating seizures.

Specific management

Cardiac monitoring is essential if a significant ingestion has taken place. The duration of monitoring depends on clinical progress but is seldom required beyond 24 hours after ingestion. All antiarrhythmic drugs are arrhythmogenic and should therefore be avoided if at all possible, as the patient already has a significant cardiotoxic problem. In particular, the class Ia agents (quinidine, procainamide and disopyramide) are contraindicated.

Sodium bicarbonate 50 ml of 8.4% i.v. (1 mmol/kg for a child) should be given intravenously (even in the absence of acidosis) to all patients with QRS interval prolongation, arrhythmias or hypotension. Give repeated doses by bolus, aiming to keep the pH between 7.45 and 7.55. Sodium bicarbonate acts by increasing extracellular sodium concentrations and by increasing pH. If a patient requires ventilatory support, hyperventilation will reverse mild acidosis and induce mild respiratory alkalosis.

If multiple arrhythmias occur, particularly if there is evidence of atrioventricular block, a transvenous pacing wire is required (p. 20). If ventricular tachycardia occurs and a pacing wire is not *in situ*, 50–100 ml of 8.4% sodium bicarbonate should be given and then lignocaine (100 mg i.v. for an adult). Atenolol or esmolol may be of use in SVTs resulting in haemodynamic compromise (p. 18). Cardiotoxicity usually disappears after 24 hours. If arrest occurs, do not give up too early – patients have survived after at least an hour of chest compressions. 10 mg of i.v. glucagon has been used for adults with some success for resistant hypotension.

Elimination methods: peritoneal dialysis, haemodialysis and charcoal haemoperfusion are ineffective.

Recovery phase: restlessness, jerking movements, chatting and plucking at the bedclothes are common. Patients may hallucinate. Patients in this phase are not fit for discharge. Sudden death occurring several days after apparent recovery has been reported rarely, but only in patients with evidence of ongoing cardiotoxicity within 24 hours of death.

Further reading

Boehnert MT, Lovejoy FH. Value of the QRS duration versus the serum drug level in predicting seizures and ventricular arrhythmias after an acute overdose of tricyclic antidepressants. NEJM 1985; 313: 474–479.

Buckley NA, O'Connell DL, Whyte IM, Dawson AH. Interrater agreement in the measurement of QRS interval in tricyclic antidepressant overdose: implications for monitoring and research. Ann Emerg Med 1996; 28: 515–519.

Pellinen TJ, Farkkila M, Heikkila J et al. Electrocardiographic and clinical features of tricyclic antidepressant intoxication. A survey of 88 cases and outlines of therapy. Ann Clin Res 1987; 17: 12–17.

Wolfe TR, Caravati EM, Rollins DE. Terminal 40-ms frontal plane QRS axis as a marker for tricyclic antidepressant overdose. Ann Emerg Med 1989; 18: 348–351.

Henry JA. Epidemiology and relative toxicity of antidepressant drugs in overdose. Drug Saf 1997; 16: 374–390.

McCabe JL, Cobaugh DJ, Menagazzi JJ, Fata J. Experimental tricyclic antidepressant toxicity: a randomised, controlled comparison of hypertonic saline solution, sodium bicarbonate and hyperventilation. Ann Emerg Med 1998; 32: 329–333.

Harrigan RA, Brady WJ. ECG abnormalities in tricyclic antidepressant ingestion. Am J Emerg Med 1999; 17: 387–393.

VALPROATE

Valproate is used in the treatment of absence seizures, predominantly in children, and as an adjunct in multiple seizure types.

Clinical features

The half-life is 7–15 hours in healthy volunteers, with plasma concentrations peaking 1–4 hours after dosing; the half-life is prolonged in overdose and may be up to 20–24 hours. Most overdoses follow a benign course, with nausea, mild drowsiness and confusion. Coma can occur if more than 20 mg/kg body weight is ingested. Occasionally, delayed onset cerebral oedema occurs and this resolves with supportive management. Myoclonic movements and asterixis have also rarely been reported.

> Warning! Unlike other anticonvulsant overdoses, dysarthria, nystagmus and ataxia are not features of valproate poisoning.

Essential investigations

Check U&Es, calcium and glucose as hypernatraemia, hypoglycaemia and hypocalcaemia have been reported. There is very little correlation between depth of coma or seizures and free or total serum valproate concentrations and so valproate assays are of little value, except perhaps to confirm the drug ingested.

Supportive care

In the vast majority of cases, supportive management is all that is necessary to ensure complete recovery. Correct the metabolic abnormalities if present. The drug is rapidly absorbed and therefore gastric lavage within 1 hour may be of little value. Activated charcoal (p. 10) can be given within 1 hour of ingestion but is of unproven efficacy. Maintenance of good (2–3 L/day) urine output is recommended. Recovery usually occurs within 24–72 hours. If the patient is comatose, the airway must be protected and ventilation is necessary. Seizures should be treated with i.v. diazepam (0.1–0.2 mg/kg).

Specific measures
No studies are available to support the use of forced diuresis, haemodialysis, peritoneal dialysis or haemoperfusion in massive valproate overdosage. If an elimination method is required haemodialysis is probably the best, but does not necessarily improve outcome.

Further reading
Jones AL, Proudfoot AT. Features and management of poisoning with modern drugs used to treat epilepsy. Q J Med 1998; 91: 325–332.

VIAGRA: see SILDENAFIL

VIGABATRIN

Used for complex partial seizures with or without secondary generalisation. Often used as an adjunct when monotherapy has failed.

Clinical features
Doses of 10 g per day have been ingested by adults without serious effects. Vertigo and tremor followed ingestion of 14 g/day for 3 days and recovery was complete. Drowsiness and coma have been reported after an overdose of 30 g with 250 mg of dipotassium chlorazepate with complete recovery in 4 days. Myoclonic jerks and psychosis have been rarely reported.

Essential investigations
U&Es. Measurement of serum drug concentration does not guide management, but confirms ingestion if this is in doubt.

Supportive care
Gastric lavage should be considered if more than 12 g has been taken by an adult, or 3 g by a child, within 1 hour. Activated charcoal should be given if the patient presents within 1 hour of ingestion, though is of unproven efficacy (p. 10).

Specific measures
None.

Further reading
Jones AL, Proudfoot AT. Features and management of poisoning with modern drugs used to treat epilepsy. Q J Med 1998; 91: 325–332.

VITAMINS

Children commonly ingest multivitamin preparations. Vitamins A and D may cause toxicity, but this is much more likely after chronic overdose rather than after a single acute overdose.

Warning! Some vitamin preparations contain iron which is a hazard (see p. 54).

Vitamin A: acute ingestion of 12 000 IU/kg body weight can cause toxicity. However, most multivitamin preparations contain 2 500–5 000 units per capsule and so a very large number need to be ingested to cause toxicity. Large overdoses can cause nausea, vomiting, drowsiness, dry peeling skin and more rarely signs of increased intracranial pressure (headache, blurred vision, papilloedema) and liver damage.

Acute overdosage with **vitamin D** is unlikely to cause toxicity but chronic excess causes hypercalcaemia.

Chronic excess of pyridoxine (**vitamin B6**) can cause peripheral neuropathy. Acute overdose with vitamin tablets does not require anything other than supportive measures unless iron has been ingested in toxic amounts (p. 55).

WARFARIN AND SUPERWARFARINS

Warfarin is widely used in clinical medicine as an anticoagulant. There are also many different warfarin-like rodenticides in and around the home: generally these are small wheat grains, usually dyed a bright colour (e.g. blue, red, green) as a warning. The colour used does not necessarily aid identification of the active ingredient. Liquids, which are diluted before use, and paste blocks, are less common. Although warfarin-containing rodenticides are still available, the development of warfarin resistance in rodents has led to the introduction of second generation 'superwarfarin' (or long-acting) anticoagulants: brodifacoum, bromadialone, chlorophacinone, coumatetralyl, difenacoum, diphacinone and flocoumafen. Concentrations used in solid preparations are usually 0.005% or less for the long-acting anticoagulants, 0.01% for warfarin.

Clinical features

Following a large acute ingestion, inhibition of the prothrombin time/INR may be delayed for up to 24 hours (warfarin) or as long as 48 hours (long-acting anticoagulants). The rate of inhibition is partially dose-dependant. Once prolonged the clotting time may remain abnormal for several weeks or months with superwarfarins, even with vitamin K therapy.

Warfarin is of low acute toxicity; there are no confirmed reports of fatalities. However, there have been reports of prolonged coagulopathy following acute ingestion of large doses of superwarfarins, for example 0.12 mg/kg of brodifacoum ingested by a 17-year-old male resulted in a bleeding diathesis lasting 55 days. The onset of haemorrhage could be delayed for more than 48 hours, and is manifested by bleeding gums, haemoptysis, haematuria and epistaxis. Haemorrhage of the gastrointestinal tract may result in haematemesis and melaena.

Although ingestion of domestic rodenticides can result in severe bleeding, large doses have to be ingested for this to occur. Agricultural rodenticides, or liquid concentrates used by professionals, potentially, pose a much greater hazard. In such cases an accurate trade name will be essential and a Poisons Information Service should be contacted.

Supportive care

Gastric lavage is usually unnecessary following ingestion of an anticoagulant, although activated charcoal may be given if warfarin has been taken within the last hour. Monitor the prothrombin time or INR if more than the following has been ingested:

- Warfarin: 0.5 mg/kg (or 5 g/kg of 0.01% bait)
- Long-acting anticoagulants: 0.01 mg/kg (or 200 mg/kg of 0.005% bait).

Observation is not normally necessary as the onset of clinical effects is delayed, and therefore the patient may be discharged. However, the prothrombin time must be measured at 24 and 48 hours post-ingestion: if greater than twice normal give vitamin K_1 (0.25 mg/kg) by slow i.v. injection. Further treatment must be guided by measurement of the prothrombin time; however, oral administration may be necessary for many weeks. In severe cases not responsive to vitamin K, a transfusion of fresh frozen plasma or whole blood or specific clotting factors may be necessary, and a haematologist should be consulted.

> Warning! Do not use vitamin K for correction of warfarin excess in patients with mechanical heart valves, as clotting could occur; fresh frozen plasma is a suitable alternative.

Further reading

Jones EC, Growe GH, Naiman SC. Prolonged anticoagulation in rat poisoning. J Am Med Assoc 1984; 252: 3005–3007.

Smolinske SC, Scherger DL, Kearns PS, Wruk KM, Kulig KW, Rumack BH. Superwarfarin poisoning in children: a prospective study. Pediatrics 1989; 84: 490–494.

ZIDOVUDINE

AIDS drugs are increasingly taken in overdose. Drowsiness, headache, ataxia, nystagmus and rarely convulsions occur if large quantities have been ingested. Mild bone marrow suppression may occur within 1–2 days. If a significant overdose has been taken and the patient presents within 1 hour of ingestion, activated charcoal (50 g for an adult, 1 g/kg for a child) should be given. The FBC should be monitored. Rarely convulsions occur and require treatment with i.v. diazepam (0.1–0.2 mg/kg body weight).

OTHER TOXINS

ACIDS

Weak acids (e.g. citric or acetic acid) generally do not cause corrosive damage on ingestion but are irritant. Strong acids (e.g. sulphuric, nitric, hydrochloric acids), however, are corrosive. (For hydrofluoric acid see p. 99). Acids cause coagulative necrosis, whereas alkalis cause liquifactive necrosis. The major corrosive effect of acids is on the stomach, where injury occurs most commonly along the lesser curve. Compared to alkalis, acids produce less localised injury to the oesophagus when ingested. Strong acids are also respiratory irritants and aspiration can cause mucosal inflammation, pulmonary oedema and pneumonitis.

Clinical features
Ingestion of strong acids results in an immediate burning pain in the mouth, pharynx and epigastrium, sometimes with swelling of the lips, and also, vomiting, haematemesis, salivation, ulcerative mucosal burns, dyspnoea, dysphagia and epigastric pain.

> Warning! Oesophageal or gastric damage may occur even if mouth burns are not apparent.

In severe cases there may also be metabolic acidosis, hypotension, acute renal failure, disseminated intravascular coagulation, liver damage and gastrointestinal haemorrhage or perforation. Oesophageal stricture and pyloric stenosis may develop after 2–3 weeks. Aspiration of the acid may result in pulmonary oedema and respiratory distress.

Acids on the skin can cause a variety of injuries including erythema, blistering and penetrating ulcers. However, acids cause coagulative necrosis and this often limits the depth of penetration.

Acids in the eye can result in severe corrosive injury.

Supportive care
Ingestion of weak acids requires only oral fluids, but admission to hospital is advisable for observation in all cases of ingestion of strong acids, even if diluted.

> Warning! Gastric lavage is contraindicated.

For potentially serious cases, who have ingested strong acid within 1 hour of presentation, consider aspiration of the stomach contents using a nasogastric tube.

> Warning! Neutralising chemicals should *never* be given because heat is produced during neutralisation and this could exacerbate any injury.
> Any patient with respiratory distress requires immediate assessment of the airway. Intubation and ventilation may be necessary.

Abdominal and chest X-rays should be performed in patients with severe pain after ingestion to exclude perforation. Give intravenous fluids for hypotension. Patients who ingest acids are usually in extreme pain and so analgesia, usually with opioids, will almost certainly be needed.

Endoscopy should be undertaken as soon as possible to assess the extent and severity of the injury. Endoscopy is contraindicated in patients with third degree burns of the hypopharynx, burns involving the larynx or those with respiratory distress. If perforation is suspected or severe hypopharyngeal burns are present, radiographic studies with water-soluble contrast media (a gastrograffin swallow) should be used instead.

The use of steroids for corrosive injury due to acids is controversial and we would not advocate their use. There is a high mortality rate in cases of acid-induced upper gastrointestinal perforation and aggressive surgical intervention is recommended if endoscopy reveals third degree burns of the stomach or oesophagus, or if the patient presents with signs of perforation.

If acid has been applied to the skin the exposed area should be irrigated thoroughly with water and treated as a thermal burn.

If eyes are exposed they should be irrigated for at least 15 minutes with saline or water and examined with a fluorescein stain. Referral to an ophthalmologist is advised if there is corneal/conjunctival damage seen on fluorescein staining.

HYDROFLUORIC ACID

Hydrofluoric acid is used in glass etching and metal extraction, refining and polishing. As well as being a corrosive, hydrofluoric acid also causes hypocalcaemia because the fluoride binds calcium. All exposures to hydrofluoric acid should be regarded seriously. A few grams swallowed or left on the skin can be fatal without appropriate management.

Ingestion of hydrofluoric acid can cause oral, oesophageal and gastric burns resulting in vomiting and burning pain in the mouth, throat and epigastrium. Haematemesis, hypotension and perforation can occur. The larynx may also be burned resulting in oedema and airway obstruction. Hypocalcaemia can cause tetany, convulsions and arrhythmias. Management is as for other strong acid ingestion (p. 98). Patients should be on a cardiac monitor and have their plasma calcium measured. If the patient has tetany, arrhythmias, convulsions, or if the plasma calcium is less than 2.0 mmol/L, give 10 ml 10% calcium gluconate i.v. repeated as necessary.

Skin exposure to hydrofluoric acid can result in severe and deep burns, which are extremely painful and slow to heal. The more concentrated the hydrofluoric acid, the more rapidly the burns develop (5 minutes for solutions >50%, but symptoms can be delayed for up to 24 hours with solutions <20%). The contaminated area should be irrigated with copious volumes of cold water (and clothing removed). After 15 minutes of irrigation calcium gluconate gel (if available) should be applied to the affected skin. If the pain persists or if the hydrofluoric acid was greater than 20% in concentration then 10% calcium gluconate should be injected around the burn. Patients with large burns should be placed on a cardiac monitor and should have their plasma calcium measured. If the patient has tetany, arrhythmias, convulsions, or if the plasma calcium is less than 2.0 mmol/L, give 10 ml 10% calcium gluconate i.v., repeated as necessary.

ADDER BITES

Adder bites are rare during the winter when the adder is in hibernation but are frequent during the summer months. Only 50% of adder bites are associated with envenomation. Adder envenomation can cause significant morbidity but low mortality.

Immediate pain at the bite site is common and local swelling occurs if envenomation has occurred; this can be delayed for up to 1–2 hours. The absence of swelling around the bite site at 2 hours excludes envenomation. Swelling rises to a peak at 2 days and may become haemorrhagic. Vomiting, abdominal pain and diarrhoea can start within a few minutes of the bite and loss of consciousness can occur early. Gastrointestinal symptoms settle over 2 days. Hypotension can persist or occur up to 36 hours after the bite. Deaths are extremely rare. However, patients may take as long as 3 weeks to recover fully.

The victim should be reassured. The bite must not be sucked or cut, and a tourniquet should not be used. All patients should be observed for a minimum of 2 hours, and the bite site should be cleaned and immobilised/splinted. Patients who are asymptomatic and have no local swelling at 2 hours can be discharged; all other patients should be observed for 12 hours. Blood should be taken for FBC, clotting, U&Es, CK and patients should have an ECG. Ensure adequate hydration; i.v. colloid may be required in patients with hypotension. In severe cases antivenom treatment with Zagreb® antivenom may be required. Features of severe poisoning indicating the need for antivenom administration include:

- Persistent hypotension
- ECG abnormalities, e.g. T wave inversion
- Elevated Creatine Kinase level
- Metabolic acidosis
- Oliguria
- Evidence of severe local envenomation within 2 hours of bite (even in the absence of systemic signs), e.g. swelling beyond the next major joint from the bite site, significant swelling of the forearm
- Leucocytosis (WCC $> 20 \times 10^9$/L)
- Any other evidence of systemic envenomation, e.g. pulmonary oedema, spontaneous bleeding, etc.

The dose of Zagreb antivenom for both children and adults is one 10 ml ampoule diluted in 20–30 ml normal saline and given by i.v. infusion at a rate of 2 ml per minute. This can be repeated after 1–2 hours if there has been no improvement.

> Warning! A history of asthma or atopy is a relative contraindication to antivenom use.
> Have adrenaline available in case anaphylaxis occurs in any patient.

ALKALIS

Alkalis are present in a number of household products (e.g. drain cleaners, oven cleaners, dishwasher products, some paint strippers) and are also used in industry. Substances include sodium hydroxide (caustic soda, lye), potassium hydroxide (caustic potash), calcium hydroxide and sodium metasilicate. Alkalis are one of the most common causes of chemical burns. Children commonly ingest household corrosive substances but usually ingest only small quantities and so severe effects are relatively rare. However, deliberate ingestion of alkali by an adult can cause severe damage.

Alkalis cause the most severe corrosive effects on the oesophagus, rather than the stomach as is the case with acids. However, following deliberate ingestion of a large quantity of an alkali corrosive effects may be seen anywhere from the mouth to the small intestine. The severity of injury is greatest where the pH is above 12, but is also dependent on the concentration of the agent, the duration of contact and the volume ingested. Solid preparations and viscous liquids are also more likely to produce severe injury due to prolonged contact.

Clinical features

Ingestion may cause an immediate burning pain in the mouth, oesophagus and stomach (retrosternal and epigastric pain), with swelling of the lips. This is followed by vomiting, haematemesis, increased salivation, ulcerative mucosal burns, dyspnoea, stridor, dysphagia and shock. Oesophageal, pharyngeal and laryngeal oedema may occur. Complications include gastrointestinal haemorrhage and perforation of the gut. Aspiration of alkali can result in pulmonary oedema and respiratory distress. Oesophageal stricture and pyloric stenosis may occur as late complications. Stricture formation usually begins to develop 14–21 days after ingestion. Most strictures become manifest within the first 2 months. Alkali burning of the oesophagus is known to increase the risk of oesophageal cancer, which can occur years after the initial injury. Oesophageal damage may occur in the absence of oral burns!

Supportive care:

> Warning! Neutralising chemicals should *never* be given because exothermic heat is produced during neutralisation and this could exacerbate any injury.
> Any patient with respiratory distress requires immediate assessment of the airway. Intubation and ventilation may be necessary.
> Gastric lavage is contraindicated.

Oral fluids may be given unless there is evidence of severe injury. Neutralising chemicals should never be given because the heat produced during neutralisation can cause further damage. In deliberate ingestion by adults, endoscopy should be undertaken within 12–24 hours of the event to assess the extent and severity of the injury. Endoscopy is contraindicated in patients with third degree burns of the hypopharynx, burns involving the larynx or those with respiratory distress. If perforation is suspected or severe hypopharyngeal burns are present, radiographic studies with water-soluble contrast media (a gastrograffin swallow) should be used instead.

Patients with grade 1 oesophageal burns may be discharged if they are able to take oral fluids. Those with grade 2 burns should be admitted and given parenteral nutrition. Intensive care is usually required for patients with grade 3 burns. A laparotomy may be required if there is evidence of severe gastric injury or the gastric pH is persistently alkaline. Give i.v. fluids to treat hypotension. Abdominal and chest X-rays need to be taken to check for perforation. Patients who ingest alkalis are usually in extreme pain and so analgesia, usually with opioids, will almost certainly be needed. The role of steroids in alkali injury is controversial but we would not advocate their routine use. Patients who develop an oesophageal stricture should be monitored for life because of the risk of malignant disease.

Skin burns: alkalis cause liquefactive necrosis resulting in deep, penetrative burns and necrosis, which can progress over several hours if the alkali is not promptly removed by irrigation. The injury may be painless and this can lead to a delay in treatment. There is also a risk of secondary infection of the damaged skin.

> Warning! The most important therapy for skin burns from alkali is prolonged and copious irrigation.

The earlier the irrigation is begun the greater the benefit. Testing the pH of the skin immediately after irrigation may be misleading. It is recommended that 15 minutes elapse before this is undertaken to allow residual alkali to diffuse up from the deeper regions of the dermis. Burns should be treated as for a thermal burn and referral to a burns unit may be required for management of large areas of third degree skin burns.

Ocular burns: alkalis can cause very serious ocular injuries because they rapidly penetrate the cornea and anterior chamber. Copious and immediate irrigation of exposed eyes is essential. Water (preferably sterile) or normal saline may be used, although other solutions can be used in an emergency, including tap water. The pH of the cornea and irrigating fluid from the eye should be monitored with universal indicator paper. Irrigation should be continued until the pH of the eye is normal and remains so for 2 hours. Pain and blepharospasm may make irrigation difficult and the use of anaesthetic drops may be needed to facilitate this. After irrigation, further treatment is aimed at preventing optic nerve damage from raised intraocular pressure and to protect the cornea from ulceration, perforation and infection. Urgent referral to an ophthalmologist is recommended for anything other than a trivial eye exposure to alkali.

ALCOHOL: see ETHANOL

BLEACH

Household bleaches generally contain sodium hypochlorite at a concentration of 5–10%. Industrial bleaches may be more concentrated (up to 50%). Bleach causes moderate mucosal irritation to the mouth and oesophagus when swallowed. When it reaches the stomach it reacts with the hydrochloric acid in the stomach and can liberate chlorine gas, but usually in concentrations too small to cause significant damage. However, if bleach is mixed with an acidic cleaning agent in the home, the chlorine gas that is released may be inhaled and cause respiratory symptoms.

Poisoning with household bleach tends to occur in children under the age of 5 who swallow only small amounts and rarely develop anything more than nausea and vomiting. However, adults who deliberately ingest large quantities or industrial bleaches may develop oesophageal ulceration, haematemesis or perforation and shock. Rarely, hypernatraemia or hyperchloraemia may occur.

If a child has ingested small amounts, giving the child milk will suffice. Severe poisoning in adults, however, requires hospital admission, i.v. fluids and endoscopy to reveal the extent of injury.

> Warning! Attempts should *not* be made to neutralise alkali with acid as the exothermic reaction will damage the GI tract.
> Do not empty the stomach.
> Charcoal is of no value.

BUTTON BATTERIES

Children often ingest button batteries, but severe cases are unusual. Most batteries pass through the gastrointestinal tract uneventfully, but complications may arise if the battery becomes lodged and causes obstruction or if the battery contents leak. There are several different types of battery and it is important to know which type has been ingested if the contents leak.

Clinical features
Obstruction is most likely to occur at the oesophageal level and with batteries that are more than 20 mm in diameter. If they reach the stomach most batteries are passed without difficulty in 2–7 days. Oesophageal impaction results in difficulty in swallowing, vomiting, haematemesis and irritability. If a battery remains impacted, corrosive damage can occur in the oesophagus.

Alkaline / corrosive damage can occur if the battery was leaky before ingestion, or opens after ingestion. The mouth should be examined for signs of chemical burns to determine whether the battery was leaky before ingestion. Burns may occur in the mouth, oesophagus or at any point in the gastrointestinal tract. This may present as abdominal pain, nausea, diarrhoea and occasionally haematemesis and melaena. Leaking mercury batteries can theoretically cause mercury poisoning, although there are very few documented cases of mercury poisoning due to this.

Batteries in the nose and ear can cause corrosive damage and potentially pressure necrosis.

Essential investigations

X-rays should be taken of the chest and abdomen (AP and lateral) to confirm ingestion and to determine whether the battery is still intact (no fuzzy margins) and whether it has passed down the oesophagus.

Supportive care

If the battery is seen in the oesophagus (or in the airway) and / or the patient has symptoms / signs of oesophageal impaction, the battery should be removed immediately by radiological techniques using a magnet or endoscopy using forceps etc. If the battery is in the stomach and is intact, the patient should be admitted for observation, ranitidine should be given to reduce gastric acidity together with an osmotic laxative (e.g. polyethylene glycol). Removal by endoscopy should be considered if the battery remains in the stomach for more than 48 hours.

If the battery is intact and has passed through the pylorus, the patient can be discharged with laxatives. X-rays should be repeated every 24–48 hours until the battery has been passed, to ensure that the battery remains intact.

If the battery is seen to be leaking on X-ray, or if the patient develops abdominal pain, vomiting, haematemesis or malaena, the battery should be removed endoscopically or surgically. A blood mercury level should be taken if a mercury battery has leaked and the patient has persistent gastroenteritis symptoms.

Batteries in the nose / ear should be removed immediately and if there is any sign of corrosive damage the patient should be reviewed by an ENT surgeon.

Further reading

Sheikh A. Button battery ingestion in children. Pediatr Emerg Care 1993; 9: 224–229.

Thompson N. Button battery ingestion: a review. Adv React Ac Pois Rev 1990; 9: 458–460.

CARBON MONOXIDE AND SMOKE

Carbon monoxide is the major cause of death by poisoning in the United Kingdom, and mortality is particularly high in those with pre-existing atherosclerosis. Carbon monoxide is a colourless, non-irritant, odourless gas. Sources of carbon monoxide include smoke from fires, car exhausts and the incomplete burning of gas fires or cookers. The risk of carbon monoxide poisoning is greater where ventilation is poor. As well as carbon monoxide, smoke produced in house fires contains a mixture of soot and organic particles together with other gases such as hydrogen cyanide. Carbon monoxide reduces the oxygen-carrying capacity of the blood by binding to haemoglobin to form carboxyhaemoglobin and impairs cytochrome oxidases. This impairs oxygen delivery from blood to tissues and its utilisation within tissues. Death may result from cardiac and neurological sequelae acutely and there are also concerns over long-term effects from acute, chronic and subacute exposure.

Clinical features

The early clinical features of acute carbon monoxide poisoning are headache, nausea and vomiting, ataxia and nystagmus. Later but still acute features include drowsiness, hyperventilation, hyperreflexia and shivering with piloerection. Central and peripheral cyanosis occurs. It is a myth that the skin is 'cherry-red'. Temporary or permanent hearing loss may occur. Some patients are disinhibited, agitated or aggressive, rather than drowsy. Convulsions, coma, hypotension, respiratory depression, ECG changes (S-T segment depression, T-wave abnormalities, ventricular tachycardia or fibrillation) and cardiovascular collapse may occur in severe cases. Cerebral oedema is common and focal neurological signs can be present.

Significant abnormalities on physical examination include impaired short-term memory, cerebellar signs (past-pointing, positive Romberg's test, and unsteadiness of gait, particularly heel-toe walking). Any one of these signs would classify the episode as severe. Rigidity, hyperreflexia and extensor plantars may occur in mild, moderate or severe cases. Carbon monoxide induced rhabdomyolysis leading to myoglobinuria and renal failure has been reported.

Carbon monoxide poisoning in pregnancy is likely to cause miscarriage or premature labour due to fetal hypoxia. Chronic carbon monoxide poisoning can also occur and gives symptoms which are difficult to distinguish from flu, i.e. nausea, vomiting, headache, lethargy, aches and pains.

Long term sequelae: Patients recovering from carbon monoxide poisoning may suffer neurological sequelae including tremor, personality changes, memory impairment, visual loss, inability to concentrate and Parkinsonian features.

Essential investigations

A carboxyhaemoglobin (COHb) concentration of blood is of value in confirming the diagnosis. However, its level is not indicative of the severity of poisoning. Normal values are up to 3–5% in non-smokers and can be as high as 6–10% in smokers. An ECG should be performed in anyone severely poisoned or with pre-existing heart disease. Anyone with significant poisoning requires arterial blood gas analysis. Oxygen saturation monitors are misleading (see below).

Supportive care

The most important first step is to move the patient away from the carbon monoxide source. Ensure the Airway, Breathing and Circulation are adequate and give supplemental oxygen as soon as possible. **Oxygen** should be given in **high flow**, e.g. 12 litres per minute through a tightly fitting facemask such as CPAP mask. It should be continued until the COHb is less than 5% and for at least 6 hours post-exposure. Sometimes 12–20 hours are required for this to take place. Unfortunately, pulse oximeters measure both carboxyhaemoglobin and oxyhaemoglobin and so a good saturation value does not give grounds for reassurance. Avoid the use of sodium bicarbonate intravenously, as this will impair oxygen release to tissues. Care should be taken not to give too much intravenous fluid, particularly in the elderly, because of the risk of pulmonary oedema. Most deaths occur in those who have arrested at the scene or who are unconscious on arrival in hospital. Monitor blood pressure. Control convulsions with diazepam (0.1–0.2 mg/kg body weight).

Specific measures

The use of hyperbaric oxygen is controversial and five randomised clinical trials to date disagree on whether it works or may even be harmful in clinical practice. The trials each have problems, which include too few patients, inclusion of patients who were exposed to other toxins in fires, and different treatment protocols. Table 3.1 lists the current indications and contraindications for hyperbaric oxygen therapy. The logistical difficulties of transporting sick patients to hyperbaric chambers should not be underestimated.

TABLE 3.1 When to use hyperbaric oxygen	
Indications for hyperbaric oxygen therapy	*Relative contraindications for hyperbaric oxygen*
Any history of unconsciousness	Asthma (increased risk of pneumothorax)
COHb concentrations > 40% at any time	Cardiac arrhythmias that may require immediate correction (cardioversion is not possible in a hyperbaric chamber!)
Presence of any neurological features (in particular cerebellar signs)	Claustrophobia
Pregnancy	
ECG changes	

In severe poisoning where focal neurological signs or evidence of raised intracranial pressure are persistent, give mannitol (1 g/kg i.v. over 20 minutes), to prevent or reduce cerebral oedema.

Further reading

Ducasse JL, Celsius P, Marc-Vergnes JP. Non-comatose patients with acute carbon monoxide poisoning: hyperbaric or normobaric oxygenation? Undersea Hyperb Med 1995; 22: 1–9.

Mathieu D, Wattel F, Mathieu-Nolf M. Randomized prospective study comparing the effect of HBO versus 12 hours NBO in non-comatose CO poisoned patients: results of the interim analysis. Undersea Hyperb Med 1996; 23: 7–8.

Raphael J-C, Elkarrat D, Jars-Guincestre MC, Chastang C, Chasles V, Vercken JB et al. Trial of normobaric and hyperbaric oxygen for acute carbon monoxide intoxication. Lancet 1989; ii: 414–419.

Scheinkestel CD, Biley M, Myles PS, Jones K, Cooper DJ, Millar IL et al. Hyperbaric or normobaric oxygen for acute carbon monoxide poisoning: a randomised controlled clinical trial. Med J Aust 1999; 170: 203–210.

Thom SR, Tber RL, Mendiguren II, Clark JM, Hardy KR, Fisher AB. Delayed neuropsychologic sequelae after carbon monoxide poisoning: prevention by treatment with hyperbaric oxygen. Ann Emerg Med 1995; 25: 474–480.

CHLORINE

Domestic exposure to chlorine may occur if household bleaches are mixed with acid toilet cleaners. Inhalation of chlorine causes symptoms of eye watering, cough, hoarseness and breathlessness within a few hours. Acute pulmonary oedema can also occur, particularly in the elderly.

All but those very minimally exposed should be observed for development of respiratory wheeze or oedema, e.g. have their peak flow measured for at least 12–24 hours because respiratory symptoms may be delayed in onset. Oxygen therapy and nebulised bronchodilators should be used for those who are symptomatic. In severe cases intubation may be required for laryngeal damage.

CYANIDE

Cyanide is used in industry in electroplating, metal processing, plastics production and photographic processes. Other sources include house fires (hydrogen cyanide is produced by fires involving plastics, silk and wool) and deliberate suicidal ingestion. Cyanide is also found in plants as cyanogenic glycosides, e.g. apricot seeds, bitter almonds, cassava beans.

Cyanide is toxic by ingestion, inhalation and skin contact. Inhalation of hydrogen cyanide gas produces symptoms very rapidly and can be fatal within a few minutes; as little as 150–200 ppm (50 mg) can be fatal. Ingestion of cyanide salts (sodium or potassium cyanide) will produce symptoms within 10–15 minutes, although symptoms can be delayed for up to 1–2 hours; 150–200 mg of cyanide salts can be fatal. Cyanide salts are well absorbed through the skin. Cyanides bind cytochrome oxidases and inhibit aerobic metabolism, producing a left shift in the oxy-haemoglobin curve and a metabolic (lactic) acidosis.

Clinical features
The onset of symptoms depends on the dose, route and duration of exposure. Small exposures cause dizziness, nausea, anxiety, tachycardia and drowsiness. With larger exposures drowsiness, coma, convulsions, respiratory depression, hypotension, arrhythmias, pulmonary oedema and ultimately cardiorespiratory failure occur.

Essential investigations
Patients should have blood taken for FBC, clotting, U&E, liver function tests and arterial blood gases. A lactate is also helpful if ABGs are being checked. All patients should have an ECG and be placed on a cardiac monitor. Blood cyanide levels are rarely of use in emergency management because they cannot be done rapidly enough to guide treatment. However, a sample should be taken before antidote administration for cyanide quantification at a later stage. Cyanide levels of <0.2 mg/L are seen in normal individuals (particularly smokers), 0.5–1.0 mg/L will produce flushing and tachycardia, 1.0–2.5 mg/L will produce obtundation, 2.5–3.0 mg/L will produce coma and respiratory depression and >3.0 mg/L is potentially fatal.

Supportive care

Warning! Rescuers should ensure that they do not get contaminated.

The first step is decontamination together with resuscitation.
    The victim should be removed from the source of contamination. It is vital that rescuers do not become contaminated – if hydrogen cyanide gas or liquid cyanide are involved, rescuers should wear protective clothing with breathing apparatus. Contaminated clothing should be removed and placed in sealed bags and the skin should be washed with soapy water. Comatose patients will require intubation and ventilation and all patients should receive high flow oxygen. Metabolic acidosis should be corrected with i.v. sodium bicarbonate (1–2 ml/kg of 8.4% sodium bicarbonate).

Specific measures
There are three antidotes for cyanide poisoning – nitrites (inhaled amyl nitrite and intravenous sodium nitrite), intravenous sodium thiosulphate and intravenous dicobalt edetate. In the future hydroxocobalamin may also be used, but this is not yet available in a suitable preparation in the UK.

Inhaled amyl nitrite and oxygen may be used at the scene prior to the patient getting to hospital and is often present in 'cyanide antidote kits' in industry. An ampoule is broken onto a cloth and held under the patient's nose, or it can be given via an ambu-bag.

Once the patient arrives in hospital the treatment options in addition to oxygen and supportive care are i.v. dicobalt edetate for severe poisoning, and i.v. sodium thiosulphate with or without sodium nitrite for mild–moderate poisoning. Patients with a metabolic acidosis should be given 1–2 ml of 8.4% sodium bicarbonate.

Patients with severe features (coma, respiratory depression, hypotension, metabolic acidosis) should be treated with i.v. dicobalt edetate 20 ml of 1.5% (300 mg) given as a bolus over 1 minute followed by 50 ml of 50% dextrose. Dicobalt edetate can be associated with severe adverse effects including facial and laryngeal oedema, bronchospasm and rashes. These are more likely to occur if dicobalt edetate is given in the absence of cyanide ions or if the drug is injected too rapidly. Facilities for intubation and adrenaline should be available.

> Warning! Only give dicobalt edetate if the diagnosis is certain and the patient has severe clinical features. If the diagnosis is uncertain or if dicobalt edetate is unavailable, the patient should be treated with a combination of i.v. sodium thiosulphate (25 ml of 50%, 12.5 g) and i.v. sodium nitrite (10 ml of 3%, 300 ml).

Further antidotal therapy may be necessary with sodium thiosulphate, sodium nitrite or a single further dose of dicobalt edetate, but this should be discussed with a poisons centre.

Patients with moderate poisoning (brief episode of loss of consciousness, convulsions, vomiting) should be treated with 50 ml of 25% (12.5 g) sodium thiosulphate given i.v. over 10 minutes. This can be followed in those with more severe effects by sodium nitrite 10 ml of 30% (300 ml) given intravenously over 15 minutes.

Patients with mild poisoning (nausea, dizziness, headache) should be given oxygen and observed; treatment with antidote will only be necessary if they develop more severe features.

ESSENTIAL OILS

There are many different essential oils, including oil of cloves, eucalyptus, cinnamon, lavender, peppermint, rose, etc. Essential oils are used as perfumes and flavourings, and although their medical use is now limited, they are becoming increasingly popular in alternative remedies. Children often accidentally ingest them. They are irritant and can cause vomiting, abdominal pain and diarrhoea. They can also cause hepatotoxicity and neurological toxicity with drowsiness, coma and convulsions. Aspiration can result in a chemical pneumonitis. All cases of essential oil ingestion should be regarded as potentially serious because even small amounts can result in severe effects and children should be observed for a period of 12 hours after ingestion. Convulsions should be treated with i.v. diazepam (0.1–0.2 mg/kg body weight).

DETERGENTS

Detergents are used in a wide variety of products, including bubble bath, carpet shampoo, dishwasher rinse aid, fabric conditioner, washing liquids and powders, general purpose cleaners, shampoo, washing-up liquid and some toilet cleaners. Detergents are of low toxicity and may cause nausea, vomiting or diarrhoea, though the main risk is aspiration of the foam produced during vomiting.

In most cases active treatment is rarely required, except for oral or i.v. fluid replacement. A dose of dimethicone or simethicone (activated dimethicone) syrup will act as an antifoaming agent if foaming is a problem. Aspiration should be treated conventionally.

ETHANOL/ALCOHOL

Ethanol is found not just in alcoholic drinks, but also in many household preparations, e.g. mouthwashes and antiseptics (10–70% ethanol), 'surgical spirit' (70–90% ethanol), perfumes/aftershave (40–80% ethanol). Ethanol is commonly taken with other drugs in overdose.

Clinical features

The fatal dose of absolute ethanol is 6–10 ml/kg body weight in adults and 4 ml/kg body weight in children. A 10 kg child only needs to ingest ~70 ml of 40% ethanol (vodka/gin/whisky or mouthwash) to be at risk of severe toxicity.

The average adult metabolises 7–10 g of ethanol per hour, thereby reducing blood ethanol levels by 150–200 mg/L/hour. Children and chronic alcoholics metabolise ethanol at a greater rate.

Ethanol is rapidly absorbed and generally absorption is 80–90% complete in 1 hour. Mild effects (blood alcohol < 1.5 g/L) include impaired coordination and reaction time, emotional lability.

Moderate effects (blood alcohol 1.5–3 g/L) include dysarthria, ataxia, diplopia, behavioural changes, flushing, sweating and tachycardia.

Severe effects (blood alcohol 3–5 g/L) include hypothermia, stupor, drowsiness progressing to coma and a metabolic acidosis. Severe hypoglycaemia (particularly in children) may lead to convulsions. Blood alcohol levels of > 5 g/L are associated with coma, convulsions, hypotension and respiratory depression – respiratory arrest and/or circulatory failure may follow.

Essential investigations

Blood or breath alcohol level (less accurate) should be determined if the patient is symptomatic (see Table 3.2). However, the level required to cause symptoms is variable and dependent on the individual's tolerance to ethanol. Levels of 3 g/L are usually sufficient to cause coma in novice drinkers, but alcoholics may be awake with levels of 5 g/L.

TABLE 3.2 Interpretation of blood ethanol level	
Blood ethanol level	*Effect*
0.8 g/L	Legal blood level limit for driving in the UK
1.5 g/L	Intoxication even in a tolerant individual
3–4 g/L	Associated with stupor and coma
>5 g/L	Potentially fatal

At blood alcohol levels of >1.5 g/L, metabolic acidosis, hypoglycaemia and hypokalaemia are common and so all symptomatic patients should have U&Es, glucose and arterial blood gases. Children are particularly prone to hypoglycaemia and so all symptomatic children should have regular BMs.

Supportive care

Gastric lavage is rarely necessary as ethanol is rapidly absorbed; activated charcoal does not adsorb alcohol and so should not be given unless other toxins have been co-ingested.

Observation is recommended for at least 4 hours post-ingestion, or until the patient is asymptomatic. Protect the airway to prevent aspiration. Intubation and ventilation may be required for respiratory depression. Ensure the patient is well hydrated. If the patient is hypoglycaemic administer i.v. 50 ml of 50% and then an infusion of 10% dextrose. In a chronic alcoholic it is important to give i.v. thiamine (Pabrinex) before dextrose because of the risk of precipitating Wernicke's encephalopathy. Acidosis will usually respond to correction of the hypoglycaemia and hypovolaemia but additional sodium bicarbonate may occasionally be required.

Convulsions usually respond to the correction of hypoglycaemia. Diazepam may occasionally be necessary (0.1–0.2 mg/kg body weight i.v.).

Specific measures

Supportive care is usually sufficient and haemodialysis should be reserved for life-threatening cases. It should be considered if the blood ethanol level is >5 g/L or the arterial pH <7.

Further reading
Atassi WA, Noghnogh AA, Hariman R, Jayanthi S, Cheung SF, Kjellstrand CM, Ing TS. Hemodialysis as a treatment of severe ethanol poisoning. Int J Artif Organs 1999; 22(1): 18–20.

Hussain SZ, Rawal J, Henry JA. Gastric evacuation for acute ethanol intoxication in a three year old. J Accid Emerg Med 1998; 15(1): 54–62.

Shulman JD, Wells LM. Acute ethanol toxicity from ingesting mouthwash in children younger than 6 years of age. Pediatr Dent 1997; 19(6): 404–408.

ETHYLENE GLYCOL AND METHANOL

Antifreeze for use in car radiators commonly contains methanol or ethylene glycol. It is usually dyed a bright colour (e.g. red, blue, green) and the usual working dilution is 1 : 3 to 1 : 4. Other sources of methanol and ethylene glycol include copy fluids, brake fluids and paint removers. Both methanol and ethylene glycol are essentially non-toxic, the toxicity being due to the metabolites produced by the action of alcohol dehydrogenase. Mortality and morbidity are particularly dependent on the time between ingestion and treatment.

Clinical features
Methanol is metabolised by alcohol dehydrogenase to formaldehyde, which is further metabolised to formate, which causes profound metabolic acidosis and ocular toxicity. The dose reported to cause ocular toxicity in an adult is 30 ml, with 60 ml the usual minimum fatal dose in an adult. However much larger doses have been survived.

At 30 minutes to 2 hours post-ingestion clinical effects resemble those of mild ethanol intoxication with drowsiness, confusion and irritability. After a latent phase of anything between 6 and 30 hours (longer if the patient has co-ingested ethanol) dizziness, drowsiness, vomiting, abdominal pain and diarrhoea occur. If treatment is delayed a severe metabolic acidosis develops with drowsiness, coma, convulsions and acute renal failure.

Ocular effects develop 6–24 hours after ingestion. Patients may initially complain of blurred or 'snowfield' vision, with whiteness, spots or mistiness within the visual field. On examination, impaired visual acuity and pupillary response to light may be seen, though usually the pupils continue to react to accommodation. On fundoscopy, the optic disc may be hyperaemic and the surrounding retina oedematous. In some cases these features are followed by permanent blindness or visual impairment.

Ethylene glycol is metabolised to glycoaldehyde, which is then metabolised to glycolic, glyoxylic and oxalic acids. These acids cause a metabolic acidosis, and oxalate causes renal damage and hypocalcaemia by binding to calcium to form calcium oxalate, crystals of which appear in the urine. The usual quoted fatal dose for an adult is 100 ml, although larger doses have been survived.

Early features appear within 30 minutes to 1 hour after ingestion and resemble ethanol intoxication; these features include drowsiness, nausea, confusion and irritability. After a latent phase of 4–12 hours, drowsiness, tachycardia and hypertension occur. If treatment is delayed a severe metabolic acidosis develops with drowsiness, coma, convulsions, acute renal failure, myocardial depression and pulmonary oedema; mortality is high in patients who develop these features. Formation of calcium oxalate may lead to symptomatic hypocalcaemia with tetany, arrhythmias and convulsions.

Essential investigations

The diagnosis of ethylene glycol/methanol poisoning can be difficult because ethylene glycol/methanol assays are not widely available. Other markers often have to be used to make the diagnosis.

In ethylene glycol poisoning urine, microscopy should be performed to look for oxalate crystals; however, they are only present in 50% of cases. All patients should have an anion gap (p. 8) and arterial blood gas measured. However, the high anion gap metabolic acidosis is due to the metabolites and may take 6–24 hours to develop.

The osmolal gap (difference between the measured and calculated osmolality) should also be measured (p. 8). An osmolal gap of > 10 mOsm is significant. However, other substances can cause a rise in the osmolal gap (p. 8). A normal osmolal gap does not exclude poisoning with ethylene glycol/methanol but if the osmolal and anion gaps are both normal and the patient is asymptomatic then significant ingestion is unlikely to have occurred.

Ethylene glycol and methanol levels, if they are available, are also not without their problems. They can be useful to confirm ingestion, and if high can be used to guide treatment, but a low concentration may simply mean that most of the parent compound has been metabolised. Formate levels can also be checked in patients who have taken methanol.

Supportive care

Small, accidental ingestions by adults of dilute antifreeze probably require no treatment; however, it may be wise to recommend oral ethanol only. In all other cases, gastric lavage or nasogastric aspiration should be carried out for any amount in an adult or a child if they present within an hour of ingestion. Activated charcoal does *not* adsorb alcohols. Observe for at least 12 hours, longer if any clinical effects or biochemical abnormalities develop. Metabolic acidosis should be treated aggressively with i.v. sodium bicarbonate, and large doses may be required; electrolytes should be carefully monitored.

Warning! Symptomatic hypocalcaemia (tetany, convulsions or arrhythmias) in ethylene glycol poisoning should be treated with i.v. calcium gluconate. Do not treat asymptomatic hypocalcaemia because this increases calcium oxalate deposition in the kidneys and brain.

Specific measures

Ethanol is the most widely used antidote for methanol and ethylene glycol poisoning and acts by saturating alcohol dehydrogenase, preventing the formation of the toxic metabolites. 4-methylpyrazole (4-MP) is a newer antidote, which is also an alcohol dehydrogenase inhibitor. Ethanol is generally the antidote of choice, although there are a few circumstances where 4-MP is preferred (see below).

Ethanol therapy: while waiting for laboratory results (but after taking blood for determination of the methanol/ethylene glycol concentration or an osmolal gap), all patients who have ingested a significant amount of ethylene glycol/methanol should receive a **loading dose** of ethanol:

- 7.5 ml/kg of 10% ethanol in water i.v. over 30 mins (solutions stronger than 10% should not be given peripherally)

OR

- 1 ml/kg 100% ethanol (suitably diluted) **orally** over 15–30 mins

OR

- 2.5 ml/kg 40% ethanol (most spirits, i.e. vodka, gin, whisky) diluted with orange juice/water **orally** over 15–30 mins.

The indications for continued ethanol therapy are:

- Methanol or ethylene glycol concentration > 200 mg/L
- Acidosis (pH < 7.3)
- Osmolal gap > 10 mOsm/kg H_2O
- Formate concentration > 10 mg/L
- Urinary oxalate crystals
- Severe symptoms.

The dose of ethanol required (Table 3.3) can be difficult to predict, and because ethanol metabolism is variable and unpredictable it is important that ethanol concentrations are checked frequently in all patients on an ethanol infusion. The dose should be adjusted to achieve a blood ethanol concentration of **1–1.5 g/L** (100–150 mg/dl). Adverse effects of ethanol at these doses include nausea and vomiting, drowsiness, confusion and, particularly in children, hypoglycaemia.

TABLE 3.3 Dose of ethanol for maintenance treatment of methanol/ethylene glycol poisoning (i.v. infusions should be diluted with 5% dextrose or 0.9% saline)

Patient	Amount of ethanol needed	5% Ethanol (oral or i.v.)	10% Ethanol (oral or i.v.)
Non-drinker/child	66 mg/kg/hr	1.65 ml/kg/hr	0.825 ml/kg/hr
Average adult	110 mg/kg/hr	2.76 ml/kg/hr	1.38 ml/kg/hr
Chronic drinker	154 mg/kg/hr	3.9 ml/kg/hr	1.95 ml/kg/hr

Continue ethanol therapy until methanol/ethylene glycol are no longer detectable. If the patient requires haemodialysis, the dose of ethanol will have to be increased by up to 100 mg/kg/hr. An alternative is to put ethanol in the dialysate.

Warning! Where ethanol is given as antidote, frequent monitoring of blood levels to ensure they are adequate will be necessary.

4-methylpyrazole therapy: 4-methylpyrazole (4-MP) is also a potent inhibitor of alcohol dehydrogenase. Although it is expensive, it has potential advantages over ethanol, in particular it does not cause CNS depression and it has predictable pharmacokinetics and so is given in 12-hourly i.v. doses without the need for frequent blood monitoring. The loading dose of 4-MP is 15 mg/kg i.v. followed by 10 mg/kg i.v. every 12 hours for four doses and then 15 mg/kg i.v. every 12 hours until ethylene glycol/methanol are undetectable. The dose needs to be adjusted if the patient requires haemodialysis – this should be discussed with a poisons centre.

Indications for 4-MP rather than ethanol:

- Ingestion of multiple substances with decreased level of consciousness
- Decreased level of consciousness
- Lack of adequate intensive care staffing or laboratory support to monitor ethanol administration.

The only absolute contraindication to use of 4-MP is if the patient is on or has co-ingested disulfiram. Relative contraindications to ethanol include if the patient is on or has co-ingested metronidazole, has gastrointestinal ulceration, children under 5 years of age and patients with severe hepatic disease.

Haemodialysis: ethylene glycol, methanol and their toxic metabolites are all well cleared by haemodialysis. Haemodialysis should be considered in severe cases.

Indications for haemodialysis in methanol/ethylene glycol poisoning:

- Methanol or ethylene glycol concentration > 500 mg/L
- Severe metabolic acidosis (pH < 7.25–7.3) unresponsive to therapy
- Renal failure
- Presence of ocular signs in methanol poisoning
- Formate concentration > 500 mg/L in methanol poisoning.

Haemodialysis should be continued until the methanol/ethylene glycol concentration is < 200 mg/L and the metabolic abnormalities have been corrected. During haemodialysis ethanol/4-MP treatment should be continued but the doses will need to be adjusted as discussed above. If the patient is being treated with ethanol it is often easier to put ethanol in the dialysate.

Although less effective, peritoneal dialysis has been used and could be considered where haemodialysis facilities are not available.

Further reading

Barceloux DG, Krenzelok EP, Olson K, Watson W. American Academy of Clinical Toxicology practice guidelines on the treatment of ethylene glycol poisoning. Clin Toxicol 1999; 37(5): 537–560.

Borron SW, Megabarne B, Baud FJ. Fomeprizole in the treatment of uncomplicated ethylene glycol poisoning. Lancet 1999; 354: 831.

Brent J, McMartin K, Phillips S, Burkhart KK, Donovan JW, Wells M, Kulig K. Fomeprizole for the treatment of ethylene glycol poisoning. NEJM 1999; 340: 832–838.

Jacobsen D, McMartin KE. Methanol and ethylene glycol poisonings: mechanism of toxicity, clinical course, diagnosis and treatment. Med Toxicol 1986; 1: 309–334.

FLUORIDE TABLETS

These tablets are used to help prevent dental caries. Many children develop little more than vomiting and nausea if excess is taken. Rarely, more than 30 mg sodium fluoride/kg body weight binds calcium causing tetany, convulsions and ventricular arrhythmias. Coma can occur due to hypoxia and a direct toxic effect on the CNS. Respiratory and acute renal failure may follow.

Ingestion of less than 10 mg/kg body weight requires treatment with milk alone to absorb the fluoride. Ingestion of more than 20 mg/kg body weight requires hospital admission for additional observation and supportive care. A patient with serious fluoride poisoning should have their cardiac rhythm monitored and convulsions should be treated with i.v. diazepam (0.1–0.2 mg/kg body weight).

HYDROFLUORIC ACID: see ACID

ISOPROPANOL (ISOPROPYL ALCOHOL)

This is found in window cleaners, antiseptics, cosmetics such as hairspray and nail polish, and in some antifreeze/screen washes. It is rapidly absorbed both by inhalation and ingestion and can also be absorbed through the skin.

Ingestion can cause gastrointestinal irritation with burning in the mouth and throat, epigastric pain, and nausea and vomiting. Poisoning by any route causes intoxication similar to ethanol with slurred speech, ataxia and drowsiness. Isopropanol is also metabolised to acetone which will be smelt on the breath; acetone also causes flushing and headaches and worsens CNS effects. Large ingestions can be associated with coma, convulsions, hypotension, arrhythmias and acute renal failure. Management is supportive – protect the airway and ventilate if necessary. In severe cases with features such as acute renal failure or prolonged coma, haemodialysis may be necessary but in practice this is rarely necessary.

LEAD

Population blood lead concentrations have fallen by up to 80% in the last twenty years. However, cases of lead poisoning continue to occur. Lead poisoning may result from chronic occupational exposure (e.g. lead smelters, battery manufacturers, painter/decorators) or chronic exposure in the home. Common sources in the home include leaded paint (particularly in pre-war homes), dust and soil contaminated with lead, water contaminated by lead pipes or lead solder, and food contaminated by lead soldered cans or lead contaminated ceramics. Lead poisoning has also been reported from the use of surma cosmetics, following ingestion of a lead foreign body, due to lead gunshot pellets and following the use of traditional remedies such as ayruvedic medicines. Lead is poorly absorbed through the skin. Adults absorb about 10% and children about 40–50% of orally ingested lead. Sanding or heat removal of leaded paint can also result in significant absorption.

Clinical effects
Lead poisoning can cause many different clinical effects in different systems:

- Gastrointestinal – colicky abdominal pain, anorexia, nausea and constipation occur at blood lead concentrations $>450–600\,\mu g/L$. Severe abdominal pain mimicking an acute abdomen can rarely occur.
- Haematological – lead affects lead cell enzymes and blood lead concentrations $>450\,\mu g/L$ can be associated with a microcytic anaemia (basophilic stippling may be seen on the blood film).
- Neurological
  — Severe lead poisoning in children (blood lead $>750–1000\,\mu g/L$) can be associated with encephalopathy (delirium, ataxia, coma, convulsions).
  — Moderate lead poisoning (blood lead $450–750\,\mu g/L$) can be associated with lethargy, irritability, poor concentration and headache. Chronic poisoning can be associated with motor neuropathies.
  — Chronic low-level lead poisoning ($<450\,\mu g/L$) may be associated with *mild* long-term neurodevelopmental effects.
- Other – lead poisoning can also cause nephrotoxicity, hypertension and hypocalcaemia.

Essential investigations
Blood lead is the most useful indicator of lead poisoning (samples should be taken in an EDTA tube). 'Normal' blood lead concentrations are less than $100\,\mu g/L$. Patients should also have a FBC and blood film, U&E, liver function tests and calcium. Lead causes changes in red cell and urinary porphyrins but these should not be measured routinely. An abdominal X-ray (AXR) should be performed in children with lead poisoning, particularly if

there is a history of pica, to exclude ingested lead paint, or lead foreign bodies. Long bone X-ray in children with lead poisoning may show 'lead lines'.

Supportive care

Activated charcoal does not adsorb lead. If a child presents after ingestion of lead paint or a lead foreign body, and these are seen on AXR, whole bowel irrigation should be considered (p. 12).

The most important aspect of management of lead poisoning is to remove the patient from the source of lead poisoning. It can often be difficult to identify the source and it may be necessary to involve Environmental Health Services and take samples from the home.

Children with lead encephalopathy should be admitted to paediatric intensive care and further advice sought from a poisons centre.

Warning! Lumbar puncture should not be performed in children with lead encephalopathy.
The most important thing in treating lead poisoning is to find the source and prevent further exposure.

Specific measures

There are two agents used for chelation therapy in lead poisoning – intravenous EDTA (sodium calcium edetate) and oral DMSA (2,3-dimercaptosuccinic acid). Other older agents (BAL (British Anti-Lewsite) and penicillamine) are rarely used for the treatment of lead poisoning now.

Chelation therapy should be discussed with a poisons centre. In general children with a blood lead concentration > 450 μg/L should be treated with chelation therapy. Children with encephalopathy or a blood lead concentration > 750 μg/L require admission for urgent chelation therapy and further advice should be sought from a poisons centre (p. 138). Chelation therapy should also be considered in symptomatic adults, but often removal from further exposure is all that is required in adults with lead poisoning.

Further reading

Committee on Drugs, American Academy of Pediatrics. Treatment guidelines for lead exposure in children. Pediatrics 1994; 96: 155–160.

Angle CR. Childhood lead poisoning and its treatment. Ann Rev Pharmacol Toxicol 1993; 32: 409–434.

MERCURY

Mercury is available in inorganic, organic and elemental forms. The patterns and severity are dependent both on the form of mercury and the route of exposure.

TABLE 3.4   Mercury – absorption and toxicity

Type of Mercury	Absorption		Toxicity		
	Inhalation	Ingestion	Gastrointestinal	Renal	Neurological
Elemental Mercury (liquid)	Not applicable	No	No	No	No
Elemental Mercury (vapour)	+ + +	Not applicable	No	Rare	Yes
Inorganic Mercury	No	+ +	Yes	Yes	No
Organic Mercury	+ +	+ + +	No	Rare	Yes

The commonest mercury exposures are:

- Ingestion of elemental mercury – e.g. mercury thermometer broken in the mouth. This does *not* result in systemic toxicity as elemental mercury is not absorbed from the GI tract and does not cause local GI effects. No treatment or intervention is required.
- Inhalation of elemental mercury vapour – acute, high dose inhalation (e.g. mercury from a barometer broken on the floor) may produce respiratory irritation but only very rarely produces the systemic effects seen with chronic exposure (gingivitis, tremor, lethargy, hallucinations and personality changes).
- Ingestion of inorganic mercury (e.g. mercuric chloride) – this causes GI corrosive damage and potentially GI haemorrhage. Absorption of inorganic mercury leads to acute renal failure but neurological effects are not seen.

   Urine and blood samples should be taken for mercury concentrations after significant exposures (but are not necessary after oral elemental mercury ingestion) and advice on further management, including chelation therapy, should be sought from a poisons centre (p. 138).

METHANOL: see ETHYLENE GLYCOL

MUSHROOMS
MAGIC MUSHROOMS
These hallucinogenic mushrooms are eaten for 'fun'. The *Psilocybe semilanceata* or liberty cap is most commonly involved from August to January. Onset of effects is usually within 30–90 minutes of ingestion with nausea, vomiting, abdominal pain, dilated pupils, visual and auditory hallucinations and more rarely agitation or drowsiness. Sedation is sometimes necessary if hallucinations and agitation are extreme.

TOXIC MUSHROOMS

90% of all mushroom-related deaths are due to *Amanita phalloides* (the death cap). Many poisonous mushrooms are available to the public, however, and people seem to show a stark lack of knowledge of them before eating them. The majority of toxic mushrooms cause a mild to moderate self-limiting gastroenteritis. The critical things to ask the patient are the interval between ingestion and onset of gastrointestinal symptoms, and whether the mushrooms were cooked. In general, the sooner symptoms start, the less toxic the mushroom, although this is clearly of no value if a mixture has just been eaten.

Amanita causes symptoms after a latent period of 12 hours – initially vomiting, severe abdominal pain and diarrhoea with dehydration and electrolyte imbalance. This is followed 2–3 days later by liver damage and fulminant hepatic failure.

If poisoning with a toxic mushroom is suspected then the patient should be admitted, preferably with samples of any mushroom types eaten. These can be identified from wallcharts or books, or by contact with expert mycologists known to the National Poisons Information Service Centres (p. 138). Management is supportive, with rehydration in patients who are vomiting or have diarrhoea. The stomach should be emptied if a patient presents within 1 hour and the mushroom type is unknown or known to be toxic. Activated charcoal can also been given up to 1–2 hours after ingestion.

PESTICIDES

Pesticides include a variety of agents that are specifically classified on the basis of their target organisms.

- Herbicides, e.g. paraquat, diquat, chlorates, chlorophenoxyacetate ('hormone') weedkillers
- Insecticides, e.g. organophosphorus compounds, pyrethrins/pyrethroids, carbamates
- Molluscicides, e.g. metaldehyde
- Fungicides, e.g. carbamates
- Rodenticides, e.g. superwarfarins (see under warfarin (p. 95) in the drugs section).

PARAQUAT

Paraquat is a herbicide used for weed control. Occupational poisoning has occurred by transdermal absorption when concentrated spray solutions have leaked from backpacks but in general it is poorly absorbed through intact skin or the respiratory tract. However, paraquat is more commonly used as a means of suicide by deliberate ingestion and has a high fatality rate. It is available in concentrated (agricultural up to 20%) and dilute (granular

2.5–8%) forms, and it is important to check which preparation has been ingested. Paraquat is rapidly absorbed from the gastrointestinal tract and peak levels are achieved 2 hours after ingestion.

Absorbed paraquat is sequestered in the lungs and undergoes a complex sequence of changes that result in the production of hydrogen peroxide and super oxide anions, which attack lipids present in cell membranes and cause cell death. An acute alveolitis develops causing haemorrhagic pulmonary oedema or adult respiratory distress syndrome. The lethal dose for an adult is estimated to be of the order of 2–4 g; therefore as little as 10–20 ml of a 20% solution can be fatal. The features of upper gastrointestinal and respiratory tract damage reflect the concentration of the solution swallowed, while the systemic features are more due to the amount ingested. Once sprayed onto crops/soil, paraquat is rapidly bound and so is not likely to be toxic.

Clinical features

Ingestion of concentrated solutions causes pain and swelling in the mouth with throat and oral ulcers. The time course, features and outcome of paraquat poisoning depend on the amount ingested and three common clinical courses are seen:

1. Ingestion of >6 g paraquat by an adult (80 mg paraquat/kg body weight) results in a rapidly progressive illness with death in 24–48 hours. Corrosive gastrointestinal injury with painful buccal ulceration, dysphagia, vomiting, abdominal pain, and diarrhoea is followed by renal failure, shock, metabolic acidosis and coma with dyspnoea and cyanosis due to pneumonitis.
2. Ingestion of 3–6 g paraquat by an adult (40–80 mg paraquat/kg body weight) results in a more protracted course but is still fatal over a period of a few days. The early gastrointestinal features are similar and are followed by progression over a few days by cough, breathlessness, cyanosis and renal failure progressing relentlessly to death. Rarely jaundice due to hepatocellular damage or perforation of the oesophagus with mediastinitis can occur.
3. Ingestion of 1.5–3 g by an adult (20–40 mg paraquat/kg body weight) results in a much more protracted course. Early gastrointestinal effects (vomiting, diarrhoea, abdominal pain, dysphagia and less commonly buccal ulceration) are followed by mild renal tubular damage with respiratory symptoms starting 10–21 days after ingestion with cough, breathlessness, basal crepitations and bilateral chest X-ray opacities. Death from pulmonary fibrosis and respiratory failure can occur as late as 5–6 weeks after ingestion.

Death in paraquat poisoning is due to critically impaired gas exchange, secondary to the pulmonary toxicity of paraquat. The development of renal failure compromises the only efficient method of eliminating absorbed paraquat and for that reason it hails the demise of many patients.

Essential investigations

The diagnosis of poisoning is usually made on the basis of the history of ingestion together with the presence of oral burns. A urine spot test should be performed to confirm absorption of paraquat: 100 mg of sodium dithionite should be added to 10 ml of 1 M sodium hydroxide and 1 ml of this solution added to 1 ml of urine – a blue-green colour indicates a positive result. A negative test within 4 to 6 hours indicates that not enough has been absorbed to cause problems and is of great reassurance value in cases of accidental inhalation or alleged ingestion.

The prognosis for an individual who has ingested paraquat can be predicted from a nomogram that relates plasma paraquat concentrations at given times after ingestion to the probability of survival (see Table 3.5). Patients who have a positive urine spot test should therefore have a blood sample taken for plasma paraquat; the assay is available in the UK at Zeneca Central Toxicology Laboratory and the Birmingham Centre of the National Poisons Information Service (see p. 138 for contact telephone number). Patients whose plasma paraquat concentrations are below the levels given in Table 3.5 at the times indicated are likely to survive. Patients whose plasma paraquat concentrations are above the levels given in Table 3.5 have a very poor prognosis, regardless of treatment, and therefore should be kept as comfortable as possible and their families given appropriate emotional support and counselling.

TABLE 3.5 Plasma paraquat concentrations as predictors of poor outcome

Time after ingestion (hours)	Plasma paraquat (mg/L)
4	2.0
5	0.8
6	0.6
7	0.48
8	0.33
10	0.29
12	0.23
15	0.17
20	0.12
24	0.10

Supportive care

Activated charcoal should be given if the patient presents within 1 hour of ingestion. There is a range of treatment options available for patients whose plasma paraquat concentrations lie below the survival line, but the efficacy of each is unproven and cases should be discussed with a poisons centre (p. 138). Symptomatic measures include anti-emetics, mouthwashes, analgesics and rigorous rehydration to replace gastrointestinal fluid losses. Palliative care is the best approach in patients with plasma paraquat concentrations above the survival line.

> **Warning!** Experimentally, supplemental oxygen has been shown to enhance paraquat toxicity and so it is probably best avoided.

It is doubtful if elimination techniques such as forced diuresis, dialysis, or haemoperfusion have any role; however, confirmed cases of paraquat poisoning should be discussed with a poisons centre.

Further reading

Vale JA, Meredith TJ, Buckley BM. Paraquat poisoning: clinical features in immediate general management. Human Toxicol 1987; 6: 41–71.

Proudfoot AT, Stewart MS, Levitt T, Widdop B. Paraquat poisoning: significance of plasma paraquat concentrations. Lancet 1979; 18: 330–332.

CHLORATES

Sodium chlorate is found in some weedkillers and other chlorate salts are used in dye production. Chlorates are powerful oxidising agents and highly toxic if ingested. The fatal dose for an adult can be as little as 20 g. Serious chlorate poisoning is rare and results from deliberate ingestion, but accidental cases have been reported as it can look similar to sugar and has been added to tea.

Clinical features

Early features of acute poisoning include nausea and vomiting, diarrhoea and abdominal pain. Methaemoglobinaemia (see p. 21) is common and massive intravascular haemolysis with haemoglobinaemia, jaundice and acute renal failure can occur.

Supportive care

Gastric lavage should be carried out if the patient presents within 1 hour of ingestion and administration of activated charcoal is recommended. The haemoglobin, haematocrit and plasma potassium concentrations will need to be monitored.

Specific measures

Methylene blue (1–2 mg/kg body weight by slow intravenous injection, see p. 22) is usually advised for methaemoglobinaemia exceeding 30%, but its efficacy has been questioned and there are concerns that its use could lead to production of chlorides and further methaemoglobin production.
Transfusion may be required to replace the oxygen carrying capacity of blood lost from haemolysis but is not an effective treatment for methaemoglobinaemia. Haemodialysis removes chlorate and may also be required for treatment of renal failure.

CHLOROPHENOXYACETATE HERBICIDES

Chlorophenoxyacetate herbicides are widely used by farmers and the public. They are popularly known as 'hormone' weedkillers.
2,4-D (2,4-dichlorophenoxyacetic acid) is the most widely used agent in this class; others include dichloroprop, mecoprop and 2,4,5-T (trichlorophenoxyacetic acid).

Clinical features
The oral dose of 2,4-D required to elicit symptoms is 50–60 mg/kg body weight. Ingestion causes burning of the mouth and throat, nausea, vomiting, diarrhoea and abdominal pain, with facial flushing and profuse sweating. Headache, dizziness, hyperthermia and hypertension may also be features. More serious poisoning is associated with muscle weakness, CNS depression with prolonged coma, rhabdomyolysis, respiratory insufficiency secondary to muscle weakness and pulmonary oedema. Renal injury with albuminuria and oliguria has been observed. Peripheral neuropathies begin several hours to 1 month after exposure and can progress to severe pain and paralysis. Recovery can be incomplete even after several years; however, the neuropathies may relate to a contaminant rather than the chlorophenoxyacetate herbicide itself.

Essential investigations
An HPLC method is available to confirm ingestion or a diagnosis of acute poisoning with these herbicides (2,4-D, dichloroprop, 2,4,5-T, mecoprop, etc.). Other laboratory abnormalities include hypoglycaemia, hypocalcaemia and metabolic acidosis.

Supportive care
Gastric lavage should be carried out if ingestion has occurred within the previous 1 hour. Ventilation may be required in patients with coma or respiratory muscle weakness. Renal function, acid-base status, blood glucose and calcium concentration should be measured in severe cases and corrected.

Specific measures
Fortunately, although there is no antidote, the elimination of 2,4-D, dichloroprop and mecoprop can be considerably enhanced, shortening the duration of poisoning, **by alkalinising the urine** (see p. 14). Urinary alkalinisation is ineffective with other chlorophenoxyacetates but these compounds can be removed by haemodialysis, which should be considered for patients with serious chlorophenoxy herbicide poisoning.

ORGANOPHOSPHORUS INSECTICIDES

Organophosphorus compounds were initially developed as chemical warfare agents. Although they have numerous complex actions their principal effect is inhibition of cholinesterase enzymes, particularly acetylcholinesterase (AChE). This leads to accumulation of acetylcholine at muscarinic receptors (cholinergic effector cells), nicotinic receptors (skeletal neuromuscular junction and autonomic ganglia) and in the central nervous system. Organophosphorus compounds are well absorbed by ingestion, inhalation and through the skin. The onset, severity and duration of poisoning is dependent on the route of exposure and the agent involved. The onset of clinical effects is usually within 1–2 hours, but can be as early as 5 minutes after exposure, or be delayed for up to 12 hours.

Clinical features

Features of acute ingestion include muscarinic effects (vomiting, abdominal pain, diarrhoea, miosis, sweating, hyper-salivation and dyspnoea due to bronchoconstriction and excessive bronchial secretions), nicotinic effects (muscle fasciculations, tremor and later weakness) and CNS effects (anxiety, headache, loss of memory, drowsiness and coma). Although bradycardia would be predicted from the mechanism of action, tachycardia occurs in about one third of cases. Later, flaccid muscle paralysis with paralysis of limb muscles, respiratory muscles and sometimes extra-ocular muscles occurs. Respiratory muscle paralysis, bronchial constriction and presence of copious respiratory secretions contribute to respiratory failure, but depression of respiratory drive is probably the single most important factor and respiratory complications are the major cause of death in severely poisoned patients. Coma is present in severely poisoned patients; rarely hyperglycaemia, complete heart block and arrhythmias may occur.

Delayed features

A small minority of patients develop the intermediate syndrome. This is characterised by cranial nerve and brain stem lesions and a proximal neuropathy commencing 1–4 days after acute poisoning and lasting for approximately 3 weeks. Respiratory depression is a complication and ventilatory support is required as the intermediate syndrome is said to be unresponsive to atropine and oximes. The syndrome has been said to be due to inadequate oxime therapy, but the aetiology is probably more complicated.

Organophosphate-induced delayed neuropathy starts 2 weeks or more after exposure and is the result of degeneration of large myelinated motor and sensory fibres. An initial flaccidity and muscle weakness in the arms and legs gives rise to a clumsy shuffling gait and is followed later by spasticity, hypertonicity, hyperreflexia and clonus. In many patients recovery is limited to the arms and hands, and damage to lower extremities such as foot drop is permanent. Not all organophosphorus compounds cause delayed neuropathy and those that do have been phased out in most developed countries.

Essential investigations

In general, clinical features are more helpful than red cell cholinesterase measurements in determining the severity of intoxication and prognosis. There is wide inter-individual variation in cholinesterase activity; however, there is a rough correlation between cholinesterase activity and clinical effects (~ 50% cholinesterase activity in subclinical poisoning, 20–50% activity in mild poisoning and less than 10% of normal cholinesterase activity in severe poisoning). An ECG should be carried out in all OP poisoned patients, and U&Es and glucose should also be monitored.

Supportive care
The management of acute organophosphorus poisoning includes clearing the airway, ensuring adequate ventilation and giving high flow oxygen. For dermal exposure, remove soiled clothing (and place it in double sealed bags) and wash the skin thoroughly with soap and water.

> **Warning!** Do not become contaminated yourself.
> Wear protective clothing.

If the compound has been ingested, gastric lavage may be undertaken within an hour of ingestion followed by activated charcoal (50 g for an adult, 1 g/kg in a child) down the tube. If possible, it is wise to confirm diagnosis by measuring AChE activity, preferably both in red blood cells and plasma. Patients who are severely poisoned with organophosphorus compounds should be managed in an intensive care unit. Convulsions and twitching should be controlled with intravenous diazepam (0.1–0.2 mg/kg), which may also have additional beneficial effects.

Atropine (2 mg intravenously for an adult, 0.02 mg/kg body weight for a child) reduces bronchorrhoea, bronchospasm, salivation and abdominal colic, and should be repeated every 10 minutes until signs of atropinisation (flushed red skin, tachycardia, dilated pupils and dry mouth) develop. Up to 30 mg of atropine or more may be required in the first 24 hours and the drug may have to be continued for a prolonged period.

Specific measures
Cholinesterase reactivators, such as the oximes pralidoxime (P2S) and obidoxime (toxogonin) are helpful if given before the organophosphorus–cholinesterase enzyme complex 'ages'. In the UK, pralidoxime should be given in addition to atropine to every symptomatic patient and the dose is 30 mg/kg of body weight by slow intravenous injection. Clinical improvement (cessation of convulsions and fasciculation, improved muscle power and recovery of consciousness) usually occurs within 20–30 minutes. The need for further therapy is guided by clinical improvement together with monitoring of cholinesterase activity. If necessary, further doses of pralidoxime can be given 4–6-hourly or by continuous infusion (8 mg/kg body weight/hour). Side effects are seen at high doses or rates of administration (more than 500 mg/minute). They include tachycardia, muscular rigidity, neuromuscular blockade, hypertension and laryngospasm.

Haemoperfusion and haemodialysis are of no benefit.

PYRETHRINS AND PYRETHROIDS

The synthetic pyrethroids are the newest major class of insecticides. Pyrethrins are naturally occurring insecticides derived from the chrysanthemum. Acute human poisoning due to these insecticides is rare; however, they can cause skin and upper-airway irritation. They are poorly absorbed from the GI tract, skin and following inhalation, and so very large doses are necessary to produce systemic effects.

Clinical features

Use indoors and in enclosed spaces has produced toxicity. The characteristic feature is cutaneous paraesthesia or a stinging or burning sensation on the skin. These are most likely to occur after exposure to products containing the alpha-cyanose substituent, deltamethrin, cypermethrin or fenvalerate. They are noticed several hours after exposure and may last from 12–18 hours. Contact dermatitis may also occur.

Spills on the head, face and eyes result in pain, lacrimation, photophobia and oedema of the eyelids. Inhalation causes breathlessness, nausea, headaches and irritability. Allergic reactions to pyrethroids are well documented and one fatal case due to bronchospasm has been reported after inhalation of a pyrethroid shampoo.

Ingestion of pyrethroids causes epigastric pain, nausea and vomiting, headache, dizziness, fatigue, chest tightness, blurred vision, paraesthesia and palpitations. Coma, convulsions and pulmonary oedema are the most serious consequences of ingestion, but are rare and only occur in very severe cases after ingestion of large quantities.

Supportive care

Symptomatic and supportive care is all that can be offered for the treatment of serious poisoning. Washing the skin may paradoxically make the skin irritation worse and is best avoided.

CARBAMATE INSECTICIDES

Carbamate insecticides inhibit a number of tissue esterases, in particular cholinesterase enzymes, particularly acetylcholinesterase (AChE). They function very similarly to organophosphorus compounds (p. 124) but their action is of much shorter duration, as the carbamate/cholinesterase complex dissociates spontaneously with a half-life of the order of 30–40 minutes.

Since carbamate insecticides act in the same way as organophosphorus compounds, the features of poisoning are similar but not usually so severe. However, deaths have been reported. Delayed neurotoxicity has been reported following acute exposure to carbamate insecticide, particularly sensory loss and weakness in arms and legs accompanied by peripheral axonal neuropathy.

The management of acute carbamate insecticide poisoning is identical to that for organophosphorus poisoned patients, with the exception that rapid recovery tends to occur with supportive therapy alone (including atropine) and the use of oximes is unnecessary (because carbamate poisoning is usually self-limiting) and may even be detrimental. In severe carbamate poisoning atropine may be given intravenously in frequent small doses (0.5–1.0 mg i.v. for an adult) until signs of atropinisation develop. Diazepam (0.1–0.2 mg/kg given orally or intravenously) may be used to relieve anxiety.

METALDEHYDE

Metaldehyde is used as slug killer.

Clinical features
Nausea, vomiting, abdominal pains and diarrhoea often occur 1–3 hours after ingestion of any amount. Ingestion of more than 100 mg/kg body weight can cause ataxia, myoclonus, convulsions, impaired consciousness and metabolic acidosis and rhabdomyolysis with hyperthermia; hepatocellular damage and renal failure can also occur.

Management
Management is supportive and symptomatic. Comatose patients may require ventilation. Diazepam is the treatment of choice for convulsions. Gastric lavage, followed by activated charcoal, should be considered if more than 50 mg/kg of body weight has been ingested within 1 hour.

PETROLEUM DISTILLATES, WHITE SPIRIT, ETC.

Children frequently ingest these products because they are readily available in most households. Some may become agitated but more often there is drowsiness which rarely may lead to coma and convulsions. Vomiting is common. Aspiration can result in severe pulmonary complications – coughing, choking, wheezing and breathlessness are the main symptoms which tend to reach their peak within 24 hours of onset and settle 3–4 days later. In more severe cases a chemical pneumonitis or lipoid pneumonia can develop. Deaths have very rarely been reported.

> Warning! Gastric lavage is contraindicated.
> Activated charcoal is ineffective.

Oxygen therapy should be used for those who are breathless, and nebulised bronchodilators may also be necessary. A chest X-ray should be carried out looking for pulmonary effects.

PLANTS COMMONLY EATEN BY CHILDREN

Most children who ingest plants in the UK develop only minor GI symptoms, and seldom more than oral fluid is necessary for treatment.

These plants are only likely to cause vomiting and diarrhoea:
African violet (*Saintpaulia ionantha*)
Asparagus fern (*Asparagus officinalis*)
Barberry (*Berberis* spp)
Beech (*Fagus* spp)
Begonia spp
Bladder senna (*Colutea arborescens*)
Busy lizzie (*Impatiens* spp)
Chinese lantern (*Physalis alkekengi*)
Christmas cactus (*Schlumbergera bridgesii*)
Clematis spp
Cotoneaster spp
Elderberry (*Sambucus* spp)
Fuchsia spp
Grape hyacinth (*Muscari* spp)
Hawthorn (*Crataegus monogyna*)
Holly (*Ilex* spp)
Honesty (*Lunaria annua*)
Honeysuckle (*Lonicera* spp)
Mahonia spp
Poinsettia (*Euphorbia pulcherrima*). N.B. Other *Euphorbia* spp are poisonous
Pyracantha spp
Rowan (Mountain ash, *Sorbus* spp)
Skimmia japonica
Snowdrop (*Galanthus nivalis*)
Spider plant (*Chlorophytum* spp)
Spotted laurel (*Aucuba japonica*, Japanese laurel)
Tradescantia spp (Wandering Jew)
Umbrella plant (*Cyperus alternifolius*)
Winter cherry (*Solanum pseudocapsicum*). N.B. Other *Solanum* spp may be
  poisonous
Yucca spp

These plants may cause severe skin reactions:
Giant hogweed (*Heracleum mantegazzianum*)
Poison ivy (*Rhus radicans*)
Poison primula, German primula (*Primula obconica*)
Rue (*Ruta graveolens*)

**These plants are potentially toxic when ingested, and further advice
should be sought from a poisons centre:**
Aconitum napellis (Monkshood)
Atropa belladonna (Deadly nightshade)
Colchicum autumnale (Autumn crocus, Meadow saffron)
Conium maculatum (Hemlock)
Daphne mezereum (Mezereon)

Datura stamonium (Jimsonweed, Thorn-apple)
Digitalis purpurea (Foxglove)
Laburnum spp
Oenanthe crocata (Hemlock water dropwort)
Taxus spp (Yew)

> Warning! Plants are commonly mis-identified, if there is *any* doubt telephone a poisons centre (p. 138) but first obtain a representative sample of the plant (leaves, fruits, flowers, etc.).

SMOKE: see CARBON MONOXIDE

SOAPS

Toddlers frequently ingest small quantities of soaps, washing powders and fabric conditioners. Only a tiny minority of children who ingest these substances develop symptoms of nausea, vomiting, abdominal pain and diarrhoea. For this group there is no specific treatment but a good fluid intake should be maintained.

However, detergent/disinfectant solutions containing 10% or more of benzalkonium chloride may cause ulceration in the mouth and oropharynx. In large ingestions coma, convulsions, muscle weakness and respiratory or renal failure can occur. Patients ingesting these products should be admitted and supportive care given.

> Warning! Gastric lavage is contraindicated.
> Charcoal is of no value.

SODIUM AZIDE

Sodium azide (NaN_3) is a white powder, and is used as a preservative in laboratory reagents and as a propellant for inflating car airbags. Sodium azide is also used in diluents in hospital automated blood counters. Sodium azide is rapidly absorbed from the gastrointestinal tract, skin and lungs and so poisoning can occur by ingestion, inhalation or dermal exposure. Onset of effects is very rapid, with recovery occurring within a few hours in mild to moderate exposures. Sodium azide interferes with cellular metabolism resulting in direct vasodilation, a severe lactic acidosis and CNS effects.

Clinical features
Clinical features include headache, nausea, vomiting, diarrhoea, blurred vision, dilated pupils, restlessness, muscle weakness, sweating, coma, convulsions and respiratory failure. Hypotension with a reflex tachycardia

and metabolic acidosis are common. In severe cases profound hypotension, bradycardia, and ventricular tachycardia and fibrillation can occur. In inhalational exposures bronchospasm and pulmonary oedema may occur.

The following are clues which may aid diagnosis:

- Patient's occupation (laboratory, munitions or petrochemical industries) and availability of azide.
- Pungent aroma to gastric aspirate/vomitus or in the vicinity of the patient.
- Development of mild toxicity (headache, nausea, dizziness) by rescuers.
- Unexplained lactic acidosis.
- The presence of sodium azide can be confirmed in the gastric aspirate/vomitus by adding a few drops of ferric chloride (10–20%). A red precipitate (ferric azide) will form in the presence of sodium azide.

Supportive management

All patients should receive oxygen and be observed for at least 2 hours after exposure. There is no specific treatment. Ventilation may be necessary.

> Warning! Doctors/nurses treating patients with sodium azide poisoning should ensure that they don't get contaminated and poisoned themselves.

STRYCHNINE

Strychnine was formerly used as a rodenticide and is sometimes found as an adulterant in drugs of abuse. It is rapidly absorbed and causes effects within 15–30 minutes. It causes skeletal muscle contraction resulting in muscle spasms that can resemble the tonic–clonic phase of a tonic–clonic seizure (however, the patient is usually awake and aware of the contractions). Repeated muscle spasms can result in hyperthermia, rhabdomyolysis and acute renal failure. Death is usually caused by respiratory arrest due to respiratory muscle spasms.

All patients should have U&E and creatine kinase measured and urine output and temperature should be monitored. Mild muscle spasms can be treated with diazepam (0.1–0.2 mg/kg) together with morphine for pain. In more severe cases, use neuromuscular blockers (e.g. pancuronium) to produce paralysis, and ventilate.

SUPERWARFARINS/RODENTICIDES: see WARFARIN

TOILETRIES

These are readily accessible in homes. Many are non-toxic and ingestion causes few symptoms. However, those containing acetone or toluene (such as nail varnish remover) or those containing ethanol (such as aftershaves, perfumes and mouthwashes) are potentially toxic and can cause central nervous system depression, renal and liver damage and arrhythmias. Only these patients need active treatment at hospital and the care is supportive. If a product containing ethanol (p. 110) has been ingested, hypoglycaemia is common in children.

TOLUENE AND XYLENE

These solvents are found in many different household products including glues, dyes, shoe cleaners, inks, varnishes, paint, paint removers and some pesticides. Exposure may occur when they are used in an enclosed area with inadequate ventilation, or may be deliberate (volatile solvent abuse). They produce CNS effects and also sensitise the myocardium to the arrhythmogenic action of catecholamines. Chronic toluene abuse can also cause renal tubular damage, cerebellar degeneration and jaundice. Early effects after inhalation of these solvents are euphoria, dizziness, nausea, ataxia, hallucinations and respiratory/eye irritation. Patients rarely present with these early features, but if larger quantities are inhaled these features can be followed by confusion, drowsiness, coma, convulsions, metabolic acidosis, arrhythmias and pulmonary oedema.

Ingestion is unlikely to lead to systemic toxicity, but can cause vomiting and diarrhoea, and aspiration may result in a chemical pneumonitis.

The most important treatment is to remove the patient from the source of exposure. Patients should be put on a cardiac monitor; unconscious patients may require ventilation. Tachyarrhythmias are probably best treated with esmolol (p. 18).

VETERINARY PRODUCTS, ACCIDENTAL SELF-INJECTION

Every year billions of animals worldwide are routinely vaccinated or given antibiotics, trace elements or other agents to protect them against disease. Vaccinations are carried out manually using multiple-dose syringes or guns, and inevitably accidents occur. Most vaccines are formulated in a mineral oil emulsion that causes a local reaction. Some also contain preservatives and diluents that can irritate. There have been near fatal and fatal consequences of accidental injection with etorphine, a veterinary opiate. Needle guards have been developed to help avoid such accidents.

Clinical features
Veterinary vaccines that contain an oil base are poorly absorbed, and pressure effects and an inflammatory reaction can cause constriction of the surrounding blood vessels. Systemic features other than those secondary to local reactions are unlikely as the vaccines are usually either killed or attenuated.

Supportive care
The key to managing injection injuries with veterinary products is swift diagnosis and decompression of the injected area, but sadly delays are

common. Because of the small volume injected, some injuries resolve satisfactorily without exploration and are simply treated with steroids. If this option is considered the patient needs observation in hospital for 2–3 days, so that decompression of the site can be urgently implemented should swelling and inflammation extend. Alternatively, immediate local decompression may be preferred with removal of necrotic fat and some of the oil. The wound should be loosely sutured to allow discharge of serum and oil into dressings and the hand elevated on a volus slab in the position of function (metacarpophalangeal joint flexion and interphalangeal joint extension). Physiotherapy should be started early. Systemic symptoms should be treated conventionally, but the possibility of zoonoses should be considered by any physician treating agricultural or veterinary workers.

APPENDICES

APPENDIX I: COMMONLY INGESTED SUBSTANCES OF LOW TOXICITY

The following substances are frequently ingested, particularly by children, and are generally considered to be non-toxic. However, oral irritation or mild gastrointestinal upset (nausea, diarrhoea, abdominal discomfort) may follow ingestion of large quantities. Specific treatment is not required and so patients/parents can be reassured.

Drugs:

- Antibiotics (*not* anti-TB drugs)
- Anti-ulcer drugs (H_2 blockers and proton pump inhibitors)
- Calamine lotion
- Emollients (E45® preparations, petroleum jelly)
- Evening primrose oil
- Folic acid
- Oral contraceptives and hormone replacement therapy
- Simple linctus
- Steroid creams
- Zinc oxide creams/lotions

Household Products:

- Cleaning Products:
    - Carpet cleaner
    - Fabric conditioner, washing powder/liquid
    - Washing-up liquid (*not* machine dishwasher products)
    - Liquid soap
- Cosmetics:
    - Baby oil
    - Baby wipes
    - Moisturiser cream/lotion
    - Solid cosmetics (e.g. lipstick, make-up)
- DIY Products:
    - Emulsion paint
    - Putty
    - PVA (polyvinyl alcohol) glue
    - Wallpaper paste
    - Wallpaper stripper (*not* paint stripper)
- Miscellaneous:
    - Artificial sweeteners
    - Birdseed
    - Blu-tack® and similar adhesives
    - Candles
    - Cat/dog food

— Chalk
— Coal
— Crepe paper
— Cut flower food
— Expanded polystyrene
— Felt tip/ballpoint pen ink
— Fish food
— House plant food
— Icepack fluid (methylcellulose)
— Matches
— Nappies
— Pencil 'leads' (graphite)
— Plasticine®
— Silica gel
— Wax crayons.

APPENDIX 2: POISONS CENTRE CONTACT DETAILS

> There is now a single number for the UK National Poisons Information
> Service: **0870 600 6266**

Calling this number will direct you to the centre responsible for your area
(individual centres can still be contacted on the numbers listed below).

Specialist teratology advice in the UK can be obtained from the National
Teratology Information Service (NTIS) on 0191 232 1525.

We have also given contact telephone numbers for a selection of other
poisons centres around the world.

EUROPE

Country	City	Number
UK (England)	Birmingham	0121 507 5588
UK (England)	London	0207 635 9191
UK (England)	Newcastle	0191 282 0300
UK (Wales)	Cardiff	01222 709901
UK (Scotland)	Edinburgh	0131 536 2300
UK (Northern Ireland)	Belfast	01232 240 503
Eire	Dublin	+353 1 8379 964
Belgium	Brussels	+32 70 245245
France	Lille	+33 0320 44 4444
France	Paris	+33 140 37 0404
France	Strasbourg	+33 388 37 3737
Germany	Berlin	+49 30 19240
Germany	Munich	+49 89 19420
Greece	Athens	+30 1 779 3772
Italy	Milan	+39 266 1010 29
Italy	Rome	+39 6305 4343
Netherlands	Utrecht	+31 302 74 8888
Poland	Krakow	+48 1221 3710
Portugal	Lisbon	+351 1795 0143
Russia	Moscow	+7 095 928 7541
Spain	Madrid	+34 1 562 0420
Sweden	Stockholm	+46 8 610 0522
Switzerland	Zurich	+41 1 251 5151
Turkey	Ankara	+90 44 33 7001

ASIA

Country	City	Number
China	Beijing	+86 1 771 9394
Hong Kong	Hong Kong	+622 141 55 23
India	New Delhi	+91 11 66 1123
Indonesia	Jakarta	+62 2142 45523
Japan	Tokyo	+81 3 7001 1415
Malaysia	Penang	+604 877888
Pakistan	Karachi	+92 21 529669
Singapore	Singapore	+65 223 5454
Sri Lanka	Colombo	+94 1 68 6142
Thailand	Bangkok	+66 2 246 8282

AFRICA

Country	City	Number
Egypt	Cairo	+20 282 8212
Kenya	Nairobi	+254 272 6770
Morocco	Casablanca	+212 0 705 30
South Africa	Johannesburg	+27 11 642 2417
Zimbabwe	Johannesburg	+263 4 79 0233

NORTH AMERICA

Country	City	Number
Canada	Ottawa	+1 613 737 1100
Canada	Vancouver	+1 604 682 2344
Canada	Winnipeg	+1 204 787 2591
USA	Boston	+1 617 232 2120
USA	Chicago	+1 312 942 5969
USA	Dallas	+1 214 590 5000
USA	Denver	+1 303 629 1173
USA	Hershey	+1 800 521 6110
USA	Nashville	+1 615 936 2034
USA	New York	+1 212 340 4494
USA	Pittsburgh	+1 412 681 6689
USA	San Francisco	+1 415 476 6600
USA	Tucson	+1 800 362 0101

AUSTRALASIA

Country	City	Number
Australia	Brisbane	+61 7 253 8233
Australia	Melbourne	+61 3 345 5678
Australia	Perth	+61 9 381 1177
Australia	Sydney	+61 2 519 0466
New Zealand	Dunedin	+64 34 797274

APPENDIX 3: SLANG NAMES FOR DRUGS OF ABUSE

A	amphetamine
Acapulco gold	cannabis
Acid	LSD or MDMA
Adam	MDMA
AKA	MDMA, MDA, MDEA
Amphet	amphetamine
Ardin	diazepam
Bart Simpson	MDMA
Base	cocaine free-base
Bazooka	cocaine
Beast	LSD
Bennies	amphetamine
Bernice	cocaine
Bhang	cannabis
Big C	cocaine
Big Chief	hallucinogens
Big O	opioids
Black beauties	amphetamines
Black tar	heroin
Blotter acid	LSD
Blow	cocaine
Blue bomb	benzodiazepines
Bluebottle	nitrous oxide
Blue caps	LSD
Blue drops	LSD
Boy	heroin
Brown caps	LSD
Brown stuff	opioids
Brown sugar	heroin
Bullet	amyl nitrite poppers
Bumblebees	amphetamines
Bush	cannabis
C	cocaine
Canasson rouge	benzodiazepines
Candy	cocaine
Cake	cocaine
Champagne of drugs	cocaine
Charas	cannabis
Charlie	cocaine
Cherrymeth	gammahydroxybutyric acid
China white	designer drugs, fentanyl or opioids
Chinese	heroin
Chinese rock	heroin

Clear rocks	amphetamine
Co pilots	amphetamine
Coke	cocaine
Crack	cocaine free-base
Crank	amphetamine
Crap	heroin
Croke	amphetamine
Crystal	amphetamine
Crystal joints	phencyclidine
Crystal meth	amphetamine
Cube juice	morphine
Dama blanca	cocaine
Dana	heroin
DCM	2,5 dimethoxy-4-methylamphetamine
Dead on Arrival	hallucinogens
Denis the Menace	MDMA
Dexies	d-amphetamine
Dike	dipipanone
Disco biscuits	MDMA
DOA	hallucinogens
Doll	methadone
Dollies	methadone
Dolophine	methadone
DOM	dimethoxymethylamphetamine
Dome dots	LSD
Domes	LSD
Dope	cannabis
Do-Do	caffeine tablets
Dose	cocaine
Dots	LSD
Downers	barbiturates
Dreamer	morphine
Dujie	heroin
Dust	cocaine, hallucinogens or opioids
Dynamite	cocaine
E	MDMA
Easy lay	gammahydroxybutyric acid
Ecsta	MDMA
Ecstasy	MDMA
Elephant	heroin
Elephant juice	opioids
EVE	MDEA
Flake	cocaine
Freebase	cocaine free-base

Ganja	cannabis
Gas	solvents
GBH	gammahydroxybutyric acid
Ghost	LSD
GHB	gammahydroxybutyric acid
Glass	amphetamines
Glue	organic solvents
Gold dust	cocaine
Grass	cannabis
Green caps	LSD
Green gold	cocaine
H	heroin
Hagga	cannabis
Happy dust	cocaine
Happy trails	cocaine
Hard stuff	morphine
Harry	heroin
Hash	cannabis resin
Hash oil	cannabis oil
Hashish	cannabis resin
Hawk	LSD
Heaven dust	cocaine
Hit	cocaine
Hocus	morphine
Homegrown	cannabis
Honey oil	cannabis
Hong Kong rocks	opioids
Horse	heroin
Horse tranquilliser	hallucinogens
Ice	amphetamines or cocaine
Indica	cannabis
Jam	cocaine
Joint	cannabis
Joy powder	heroin
Junk	heroin
Khif	cannabis
Kit-Kat	ketamine
Koks	cocaine
L	LSD
Lady	cocaine
Laughing gas	nitrous oxide

Leaf	cocaine
Line	cocaine
Liquid incense	butyl nitrite
Liquid lady	cocaine/alcohol
Liquid X	gammahydroxybutyric acid
Locker popper	butyl nitrite
Locker room	butyl nitrite
Love drug	MDMA, MDEA, MDA
M	morphine or MDMA
Magic dust	hallucinogens
Magic mushrooms	psilocybin
Marijuana	cannabis
Mary Jane	cannabis
Maui wowie	cannabis
Meth	amphetamines
Mesc	mescaline
Mexican brown	heroin
Microdots	LSD
Miss Emma	morphine
Mister Coffee	cocaine
MJ	cannabis
Mollies	amphetamines
Monkey	morphine
Morf	morphine
Morning glory	hallucinogens
Morpho	morphine
Nerve pills	benzodiazepines
Nitrous	nitrous oxide
Noise	heroin
Orange wedges	LSD
Oranges	amphetamines
Paki	cannabis
Paper acid	LSD
Paper mushrooms	LSD
Paradise	cocaine
Pearl flake	cocaine
Pep pills	amphetamines
Persian	heroin
Peyote	mescaline
Peyote button	mescaline
Pimps	cocaine
Pimp's drug	cocaine
Pink dots	hallucinogens

Pink drop	LSD
Pink Jesus	hallucinogens
Pink Peruvian Flake	cocaine
Poor man's cocaine	amyl nitrite
Poor man's speedball	heroin/amphetamine
Poppers	amyl nitrite
Pot	cannabis
Power	hallucinogens
Puff	cannabis
Purple haze	LSD
Purple wedges	LSD
Red and Black	MDMA
Red oil	cannabis
Reefer	cannabis
Resin	cannabis resin
Rippers	amphetamines
Roaches	cannabis
Rock	heroin
Rocks	amphetamines
Rock'n'roll	heroin
Rope	cannabis
Rufus	heroin
Rush	butyl nitrite
S	ephedrine, ketamine, diazepam
Schoolboy	codeine
Scoop	gammahydroxybutyric acid
Shit	cannabis
Shrooms	psilocybin
Sinsemilla	cannabis
Skunk	cannabis
Smack	cocaine or heroin
Smoke	cannabis
Snappers	amyl nitrite
Snort	cocaine
Snow	cocaine
Sodies	sodium amylobarbitone
Special K	ketamine
Speed	amphetamines
Speedball	cocaine with heroin
Speed for lovers	MDA
Spice girls ecstasy	ephedrine + ketamine + diazepam
Splash	amphetamines
Spliff	cannabis
Split	cannabis
Star spangled powder	cocaine

Strawberry	LSD
Stuff	heroin
Sulph	amphetamine
Sulphate	amphetamine
Sunshine	LSD
Super K	ketamine
Sweat	amyl nitrite
Tea	cannabis
Thai sticks	cannabis
The Chief	hallucinogens
Thing	cocaine
TNT	heroin
Toot	cocaine
Torch	cannabis
Trips	hallucinogens
Twenty-five plus	hallucinogens
Uppers, Ups	amphetamines, caffeine, ephedrine etc.
Vallies	diazepam
Vitamin K	ketamine
Wake ups	amphetamine
Weed	cannabis
White burger	MDMA
White dove	MDMA
White elephant	heroin
White junk	heroin
White lightning	LSD
White stuff	heroin
Whizz	amphetamine
Windowpane	LSD
XTC	MDMA
Yellow burger	MDMA
Yellow caps	LSD
Yellow drop	LSD
Yuppie psychedelic	MDMA
Zoom	gammahydroxybutyric acid

APPENDIX 4: FURTHER READING

TOXBASE – the primary clinical toxicology database of the UK (SPIB@ axl.co.uk).

Dollery C. *Therapeutic drugs*, 2nd edn. Edinburgh, Churchill Livingstone, 1999.

Ellenhorn MJ, Barceloux DG. *Medical toxicology*, 2nd edn. New York, Elsevier, 1997.

Goldfrank LR, Flomenbaum NE, Lewin NA, Weisman RS, Howland MA, Hoffman RS. *Toxicologic emergencies*, 6th edn. Stamford, Appleton and Lange, 1998.

Gosselin RE, Smith RP, Hodge HC. *Clinical toxicology of commercial products*, 5th edn. Baltimore, Williams and Wilkins, 1984.

Hayes WJ, Laws ER. *Handbook of pesticide toxicology*, San Diego, Academic Press, 1991.

Martindale. *The extra pharmacopoeia*, 32nd edn. London, The Pharmaceutical Press, 1999.

Proctor NH, Hughes JP, Fischman ML. *Chemical hazards in the workplace*, 4th edn. Philadelphia, JB Lippincott, 1996.

Index

UK POISONS CENTRES

UK National Poisons Information Service: 0870 600 6266

Calling this number will direct you to the centre responsible for your area. Individual centres can still be contacted on the following numbers:

Belfast	01232 240 503
Birmingham	0121 507 5588
Cardiff	01222 709901
Edinburgh	0131 536 2300
London	0207 635 9191
Newcastle	0191 282 0300

National Teratology Information Service (NTIS): 0191 232 1525